THE
Driving
Dilemma

THE
Driving
Dilemma

*The Complete Resource Guide
for Older Drivers and Their Families*

Elizabeth Dugan, Ph.D.

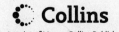

An Imprint of HarperCollinsPublishers

This book contains advice and information relating to health care. It is not intended to replace medical advice and should be used to supplement rather than replace regular care by your doctor. It is recommended that you seek your physician's advice before embarking on any medical program or treatment.

All efforts have been made to ensure the accuracy of the information contained in this book as of the date published. The author and the publisher expressly disclaim responsibility for any adverse effects arising from the use or application of the information contained herein.

HarperCollins books may be purchased for educational, business, or sales promotional use. For information please write: Special Markets Department, HarperCollins Publishers, 10 East 53rd Street, New York, NY 10022.

FIRST EDITION

Designed by Jaime Putorti

Library of Congress Cataloging-in-Publication Data

Dugan, Elizabeth.
　　The driving dilemma : practical solutions for older drivers and their families / Elizabeth Dugan.
　　　　p. cm.
　　Contents: Assessing fitness to drive—Medical conditions that increase driving risk—Driving and drugs: prescription and over-the-counter medications, vitamins, and herbal supplements—Planning to avoid dilemmas—Legal issues and license regulations—Learning to talk about change—Get talking—Resolving dilemmas.
　　ISBN-13: 978-0-06-114218-5
　　ISBN-10: 0-06-114218-2
　　1. Older automobile drivers—United States. 2. Older automobile drivers—Ability testing—United States. 3. Older people—United States—Family relationships. I. Title.

TL152.35.D84 2006
629.28'304—dc22

2006049058

06　07　08　09　10　RRD/WBC　10　9　8　7　6　5　4　3　2　1

Contents

Acknowledgments

There are many people who helped to make this book a reality. First, I want to express my appreciation for the financial support provided by the Division of Geriatric Medicine at the University of Massachusetts Medical School and the Meyers Primary Care Institute. That generous support gave me the time and resources to write this. I am grateful for the support and guidance of my division chief, Dr. Jerry Gurwitz.

I count myself fortunate to be a member of a very talented research team. I thank Vanessa Meterko for outstanding research assistance. In the early days of the project, Vanessa helped me think through the outline, conducted extensive background research, and even provided advice on what music would make me more productive. I thank Katie Dodd for her excellent research assistance. Katie tackled the daunting task of finding and compiling the information in the appendices. Her exceptional analytical skills, diligence, and energy made the project much easier. I appreciate Joann Baril's meticulous assistance with proofreading the manuscript, and thank Sherri Epstein for helping to compile and verify the state-level licensing regulations. Sherri provided important administrative and software assistance, too. The entire team carefully read draft after draft and provided constructive feedback.

I appreciate the help of Harry Margolis, J.D., and Alan Dodd, J.D., who tutored me in legal and state regulatory issues. I am indebted to many friends and colleagues who read chapters for content and clinical accuracy. I especially thank Dr. Sarah McGee, the director of education in the Division of Geriatric Medicine; Dr. Leslie Harrold, from the Meyers Primary Care Institute and the University of Massachusetts Medical School Division of Rheumatology; and Dr. Petra Flock from the Division of Geriatric Medicine.

I want to thank Dr. Tom Perls and JaeMi Pennington from the Boston University School of Medicine New England Centenarian Study for connecting me with several of their inspiring study participants. I count those conversations among my career highlights.

I am especially grateful to two experienced authors who advised me throughout the process. Stephen R. Braun, an award-winning author from Amherst, Massachusetts, provided mentoring and editing; right from the start, he encouraged me to pursue the project and deserves special thanks for thinking of the title. Jeannine Johnson, Ph.D., from the Harvard College Expository Writing Program was a great support. Despite teaching, administering a writing center, and writing her own book (*Why Write Poetry*), she gladly shared her wit, words, and warm encouragement. She deserves special thanks for helping me to make Chapter 3 understandable. Both Steve and Jeannine read every word of every draft and patiently taught me how to transform my tired academic jargon into more engaging text. The book is much better because of them; any errors or problems that remain in the text are mine, of course.

I thank my editor at HarperCollins, Toni Sciarra, for her

patience, guidance, and skill. Thanks also to Anne Cole, Shelby Meizlik, and all of the folks at HarperCollins for their contributions. In addition, I want to acknowledge and thank my agent, Jeff Kleinman, of Folio Literary Management. Jeff immediately recognized the importance of the topic and has been an energetic and effective champion of the project. The book would not have happened without him.

Many excellent sources were reviewed to develop this book; however, due to space constraints not all could be included in the final text. Please check www.drivingdilemma.com for additional, updated information. Readers should know that, when appropriate, I changed a name or minor details in a case to protect an individual's privacy.

It is impossible to fully articulate my thanks to everyone who so honestly shared driving stories, worries, failures, and successes. I remain indebted to you and even more committed to working to improve the situation.

Finally, I thank my family for their love and support—you are the greatest.

What Is the Driving Dilemma?

Even though I am a baby boomer who affectionately calls my mother "Crash," I should admit that she wasn't the inspiration for this book. Ironically, it wasn't until I was nearly finished with this project that my mother unwittingly became an example of the kind of accident that is becoming more and more common as our population ages: an older person, driving on a weekday, close to home, involved in a collision while making a left turn. Fortunately, no one was hurt in the accident, but it sure was a wake-up call for my family. After more than 50 years of accident-free driving, my mother provided an unwanted and all-too-personal case study with which to illustrate the problem facing older drivers and their family members.

One good thing to come out of my mother's accident is that I can personally attest that the steps outlined in this book work. It's no longer just an interesting topic of research for me. After her accident, my mother, my siblings, and I assessed the situation, talked over the issues that could compromise my mother's driving safety, and worked together to create a plan that works for us. The information and strategies I present can help anybody, whether you're an older adult concerned about your own driving or if you're worried about a loved one. The dilemma of figuring out if an older driver is safe and, if not, what can be done about it is common and vexing. Until now, the information you need to make sense of this situation hasn't been readily available. The research-based approach described in this book is clear, straightforward, and effective. By following these guidelines, you can not only improve the safety of an older driver, but you can also avoid the emotional land mines that can be as devastating to a family as an actual accident.

In researching this topic, I've been touched by the expressions of love, respect, and concern made by spouses or adult children for an older person who's struggling to drive safely. I've also been heartened and encouraged by the older adults I've interviewed who have faced the dilemma squarely and, whether they are driving or not, have found solutions that work in their own lives. Don't be misled—confronting a driving problem (or *a potential* problem) isn't easy or pleasant for anybody—but by reading this book, you can gain the knowledge, skills, and confidence you need to tackle a difficult family issue with grace.

The Age Wave

It's no secret that the proportion of older adults in the population is increasing. This age wave is caused by unparalleled medical and public health achievements. It is amazing to realize that *never before* in human history have *most* people in developed countries lived to old age. I hope you appreciate what an incredible development this is—on average we have an extra two or three *decades* of life compared to people who lived just 100 years ago. Gerontologists expect that older people will continue to make up an increasingly large part of the population. For example, data from the U.S. Census indicate that every day in 2005 about 6,000 Americans turned 65, but by 2015, more than 10,000 people will turn 65 each day. The overwhelming majority of these seniors will be driving. In fact, the number of licensed older drivers is expected to more than double in the next twenty years. It won't be long before one out of four drivers will be age 65 or older. Currently, about half of all women and 80% of men aged 85 and older still drive.

The good news is that older drivers are usually pretty safe drivers. Compared to younger drivers, older drivers tend to drive fewer miles per year, wear their seat belts, and rarely drive while intoxicated or get ticketed for speeding. Also, contrary to popular myth, the accident rate for even the oldest group of drivers is much lower than that of teenagers and young adults. The chart below illustrates the crash rate by age group using 2004 data from The National Highway Traffic Safety Administration.

Unfortunately, the bad news is that when an older adult *does* have an accident, he or she is much more likely than a younger

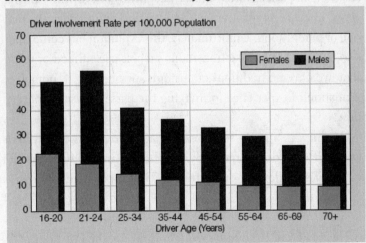

Driver Involvement Rates in Fatal Crashes by Age and Sex, 2004

National Center for Statistics and Analysis National Highway Traffic Safety Administration U.S. Department of Transportation

driver to be killed or seriously injured. Per mile driven, the fatality rate for drivers 85 years and older is *nine times* higher than the rate for drivers 25 to 69 years old. But whatever the risks of driving, older people continue to prefer it to other forms of transportation. Cabs can be expensive and difficult to hire, especially outside major cities. In addition, in many places public transportation options for older adults are either nonexistent or undesirable. More and more seniors live in the suburbs or rural areas, where public transportation is generally lacking. And even when public transportation *is* available, older adults don't take advantage of it. One study found that, in areas with easy access to public transportation, older adults report using it for less than 3% of their trips.

These trends combine to create a new—and usually disturbing—developmental milestone in life: the moment you hang up the car keys for good. Recent research indicates that most drivers will outlive their driving ability by about 7 to 10 years. Driving cessation, in other words, is fast becoming one of life's pivotal events, akin in its poignancy and logistical significance to marriage or parenthood. Unfortunately, this evolution has come upon us so rapidly that, unlike transitions such as parenthood or retirement, we have no traditions or customs surrounding it, nor a firm foundation of experience for making the passage easier on everybody.

Driving cessation is so pivotal because driving is closely associated with freedom, autonomy, youth, and an ability to care for oneself. The following quote from a 73-year-old man powerfully expresses this:

> *The day I had to give up driving was, by far, the worst day of my life. I was devastated and bawled my eyes out. I didn't know what to do—I had always been independent.*

A recognized problem with driving is likely to be a "sentinel" event in a person's life, foreshadowing other changes that threaten independence—such as a need for in-home assistance, moving to more accessible or appropriate housing, or experiencing increasingly serious health problems. Many of the strategies outlined in this book to help you talk effectively about the driving dilemma are also perfectly applicable to other age-related issues. I hope that being prepared to deal with this first challenge will help you and your family to handle other later-life issues.

What Are the Facts About Older Drivers?

Crashes. As noted above, older drivers actually have relatively low rates of accidents. But they're more likely to be injured or to die as a result of those accidents, and they recover more slowly from any injuries sustained. The most deadly type of crash, the side impact, occurs more characteristically with older drivers (particularly on left turns). Among older drivers, men are two times as likely as women to die in a crash. Most traffic fatalities involving older drivers occur during the daytime (81%) and on weekdays (72%); 75% of the crashes involve another vehicle.

Driving Modification. Many older drivers modify or self-regulate their driving behavior to avoid risky situations such as driving in bad weather, in heavy traffic, or at night. Many drivers intuitively know when to limit their driving and do so successfully. Unfortunately, however, some older adults do *not* use such self-protective measures. Adults with any type of brain disorder are less likely to self-regulate because their disorder interferes with the ability to think. Specifically, they may be unable to evaluate their driving ability or to remember to limit or stop driving. The Alzheimer Association estimates that 4 million people are now afflicted with dementia—and that number will grow sharply in coming years.

Chronic Disease. The Centers for Disease Control and Prevention reports that nearly three out of four adults age 65 and older have one or more chronic illnesses. Nearly *half* of older adults report having two or more chronic diseases. Thanks to advances in medical technology, people are living longer than ever despite such conditions. But the conditions themselves or the medications used to treat the conditions may impair driving fitness. For example, a common side effect of many medications is drowsiness, which is an obvious hazard for driving.

Age. Just because someone is 75, or 85, or 95 does *not* automatically mean they should give up driving. What matters in driving is not how old a person is, but *how well that person can see, think, and move.* Decades of biomedical research have firmly established that functional ability changes at different rates for different people. We all know people who are healthy and active well into their 90s, while others may become debilitated or die in their 50s or 60s. Age alone, therefore, is a false and unfair marker of driving ability. Chapter 1 discusses driving fitness and age in greater detail.

Giving up the keys for good can be extraordinarily difficult. It's both difficult to do and difficult to ask someone else to do. America is built for cars, and we take great pride in independence. The automobile industry invests millions of dollars in advertising to reinforce the notion that driving equals freedom and self-determination. The majority of older adults depend on their cars for nearly all their activities: medical visits, shopping, recreation, attendance at religious services, and visits to family and friends. Losing one's ability to drive isn't just inconvenient. It can be socially isolating, depressing, and even hazardous to one's health. Most of us are ill-prepared to confront this issue, are uncomfortable even bringing it up, and don't know where to turn for advice and guidance. That's why this issue is so powerful, so potentially divisive, and so frustrating.

Despite the discomfort, complexities, and challenges, however, it is vitally important to accurately assess driving ability, acknowledge the fears and emotions inherent in the issue, communicate clearly and calmly, and, if necessary, find alternatives to driving that are health-promoting and effective.

This book is organized according to the processes that an older driver or someone worried about a loved one will go through if they are concerned about driving fitness and safety:

- Assess

- Plan

- Talk

- Act

Admittedly, the organization and division of the material is a little arbitrary—because you'll have to talk as you assess, plan, and act. As a result, you might consider reading the communication section (Chapters 6, 7, and 8) before taking steps to implement the assessments outlined in Chapter 1. Assessment information such as forms to help you recognize the warning signs of driving risk, a description of medical conditions that may impair driving, and information about the impact of medications are all covered in Chapters 1, 2, and 3. Chapters 4, 5, and 6 help you to organize and use this information to develop an action plan that takes into account potential legal issues and possible barriers to effective action. Chapter 7 focuses on how to broach the issue of driving, how best to talk about it, and what pitfalls to avoid during the conversations. I include examples and exercises that can boost your confidence in talking about tough issues. Chapter 8 describes assistive devices that may extend a driver's ability to keep driving safely, action steps, and how to follow through on the plan. The appendices contain a tremendous amount of information designed to be of immediate use to you and your family.

I know that talking openly about what may be the first of many small losses due to illness or disability is not easy. The changes to you or your loved one may be distressing. Still, although this book focuses on the dilemma of driving, there may be bright spots along the way. More open communication may make your relationship even closer. I hope that the information presented here educates, comforts, and helps you and the driver you are concerned about.

CHAPTER I

Assessing Fitness to Drive

Your aunt is 86 and has just returned from a care facility where she had stayed to recover from a fall. She walks very slowly and has difficulty with stairs, but she insists she is a safe driver and hasn't had any kind of traffic accident in more than 20 years. Still, you wonder, should she be driving?

Your father is 72 and is in relatively good health, but while driving with you recently on the highway, he strayed to the left-hand shoulder, then overcorrected with a sudden jerk of the wheel. This left you frightened and him defensively arguing that it wasn't a big deal. Is he at risk?

Your mother is 75 and you've noticed that in the past couple of years she has been repeating herself—sometimes telling you the same story twice in a conversation. You notice some dings on the bumpers of her car, and a scratch on the right side. When you ask her about them, she seems surprised and says they must be from other people bumping into her car while it was parked at the grocery store. Should you be worried about her driving?

These very common situations all confront you with a similar challenge: How do you know if an older adult is fit to drive? Since age alone is not a reliable indicator, what *should* you be looking for? And, if you are an older driver, what should you be looking for in your own driving habits that might signal a need for some kind of change?

This chapter describes the most common warning signs of driving risk and gives you some tools to assess whether a real driving problem exists. Specifically, I explain what the indicators of driving fitness are, what signals a problem, how to categorize the severity of problems, how to conduct a home assessment, and what's involved in a professional assessment. Appendix 1 includes assessment forms that can be used either by an older driver for self-assessment or by a family member or friend. Appendix 2 contains forms to help you to implement changes by talking with your physician about specific functional concerns related to driving that may need some medical intervention.

Driving safety involves factors related to the vehicle, the roadways, the weather and other conditions. Above all, driving safety involves the driver. This chapter focuses primarily on drivers and on determining their fitness for driving. Although it is important to ensure that a vehicle is in proper mechanical condition, that issue is beyond the scope of this book. I'm working from the assumption that the vehicle is in good working condition. Also, other factors play a role in how safely a person can operate a vehicle: the conditions of the roads and a driver's familiarity with them, the weather, and the time of day all can affect driving safety. Obviously, all possible conditions can't be addressed here, but they should be taken into account when determining driver fitness. If you are concerned about a driver's fitness, you will want to observe his or her driving firsthand and keep a written record of your concerns. The forms in Appendix 1 should help you.

Driving Fitness and Age

At the most basic level, driving requires that we have the ability to properly **see, think,** and **move**. Limitations in any of these three key functions may signal a worrisome threat to driving fitness. Illness, age, and even significant life events can all impair your ability to see, think, and move. Significant life events, such as the loss of a spouse, may be so distressing that they contribute to physical changes that, in turn, affect driver safety. For example, the physical symptoms of fatigue and slowed thinking are common in grief. While these symptoms are perfectly normal, they can impair your ability to drive safely. See Chapter 2 for more information about common age-related changes and medical conditions that may impair driving fitness.

Contrary to what many people believe, age, by itself, does not determine driving fitness. What matters in driving are three fundamental functions: the ability to **see, think,** and **move**. These abilities change at different rates for different people. Some people in their 90s and beyond are more healthy and fit for driving than some people in their 50s or 60s. Thomas Perls, M.D., M.P.H., a professor at the Boston University School of Medicine, became interested in this phenomenon when he noticed that some of his oldest patients were some of his healthiest. Dr. Perls directs the New England Centenarian Study and is widely regarded as one of the world's leading experts studying adults aged 100 years or older. His research shows that centenarians age relatively slowly, and seem to have delayed or entirely escaped diseases associated with aging such as heart disease, stroke, cancer, and Alzheimer's disease.

I spoke with one of Dr. Perl's study participants, Ms. Nedinne Parker, aged 104. Ms. Parker is a devoted baseball fan (she roots enthusiastically for the Kansas City Royals), still lives independently, and drives once a week to her volunteer job at a local hospital. She is a remarkably healthy, active, witty woman who is still able to see, think, and move well enough to drive safely. Ms. Parker is modest about the fact that she still maintains her driving fitness. She also realizes that she has some limitations and that others may be skeptical of her driving skills. During our conversation, she quipped that she doesn't have many friends or relatives clamoring for a ride: "Well, to be honest, I don't know if I would be too quick to jump in a car with a 104-year-old gal!" She has limited herself to driving only on local, familiar roads and only during daylight hours. As a result of these self-imposed limits she has been able to maintain her driving fitness. Similarly, Mr. Edward Rondthaler still lives independently and is driving around upstate New York at 100 years of age. Mr. Rondthaler doesn't drive as much as he did when he was 80 (he drove across the country then), but he still enjoys driving around town and is doing so safely. These drivers remind us that it is not *age* but *function* that determines driving fitness.

Warning Signs of Driving Risk

If driving fitness isn't determined by age, then what are the signs of impaired driving fitness? Listed below are warning signs of impaired driving fitness based on research and guidelines developed by advocacy groups such as the American Association of Retired Persons (AARP), the American Automobile Association (AAA), and the American Medical Association (AMA).

To help you remember them, I have categorized the warning signs by level of risk into red, yellow and green. "Red" signs point to the highest level of safety risk. Having one of the red risks is a signal to immediately begin the conversation about driving and to seek a professional assessment. "Yellow" signs point to a somewhat lower, but still significant safety risk. Having one yellow risk is cause for concern, and having two or more is cause for concern and should prompt further assessment. "Green" signs point to safety risks that are usually easily corrected and, if corrected, can allow a person to continue to drive safely. If you are concerned about your driving or the driving of a loved one, *the time to start talking is now*. I can't stress this enough—being proactive and informed helps everyone. Honest and open communication is the best way to develop a plan that respects the needs, wants, and safety of all involved.

RED SIGNALS OF RISK

- *One or more auto* accidents *in the past five years.*
  A recent history of accidents is a strong predictor of future mishaps. Did the accident involve another moving vehicle? Was it a single car accident? Did it involve hitting a stationary object? The details of the accident(s) are important in evaluating the overall risk of the accident.

- *Recent* traffic tickets *or police warnings.*
  This is a serious indicator of suboptimal driving performance. Insurance companies raise their rates after a ticket or accident because such events tend to predict future problems.

- *Severely impaired vision, cognition, or mobility.*

YELLOW SIGNALS OF RISK

- *Recent near misses or close calls while driving.*
  Sometimes a near miss isn't our fault, but sometimes it is a symptom of declining driving performance. It's important to know which is the case in order to evaluate the risk for the driver.

- *Having* friends or relatives *say they don't want to ride with the driver, or having them say they don't want their children driving with that person.*

  Since people are often reluctant to speak up about their concerns for a person's driving, such expressions should be taken seriously as a sign that something is wrong. If concerns are raised, get the details and follow the guidelines presented later in this book for initiating a conversation and taking action.

- *Accumulation of vehicle dents and dings.*

  Backing into things or scraping walls or other objects may indicate vision, mobility, or navigational problems. Minor fender benders also signal that driving fitness is slipping.

- *Feeling uncomfortable, stressed, or exhausted when driving.*

  Stress and exhaustion are signs that a driver may not be feeling fully competent behind the wheel and, thus, can be a signal that driving skills are diminishing.

- *Having other drivers honk, gesture, or seem annoyed at you when driving.*

  Unless you live in a city that is famous for rude drivers, honking, yelling, or other "impolite" actions are probably a clue that a person's driving is either erratic or outside the norm, both of which can be a sign of trouble.

- *Difficulty judging gaps in traffic at intersections and on highway entrance and exit ramps.*

  Age-related changes in the eyes may impair depth perception.

- *Failing to notice vehicles or pedestrians on the sides of the road when looking straight ahead.*

  Being surprised by the sudden presence of pedestrians or cars could indicate a diminished field of view, which is vital to safe driving.

- Not seeing *lights, signs, signals, or pedestrians soon enough to respond to them smoothly.*

- *Getting* lost *more often than in the past, especially in familiar areas.*
  This could signal memory problems or other cognitive deficits.

- Trouble paying attention *to traffic signals, road signs, and pavement markings.*
  This could be a sign of a problem with the cognitive ability to divide attention and to respond to multiple cues simultaneously.

- Slow response *to unexpected situations.*
  This could signal impaired thought processes related to recognizing stimuli and attaching meaning to them or a delay in physical reactions.

- *Becoming easily* distracted *or having difficulty concentrating while driving.*

- *New or worsening* medical conditions.
  Chapter 2 explores medical conditions and driving in detail. The worsening of a condition may require adaptations.

- *Taking* medications *with side effects that can impair driving safety.*
  Many medications carry warnings about operating machinery or driving while taking them. In Chapter 3, many common medications and their effects on driving safety are discussed.

- *Not using the safety belt.*
  Forgetting to take advantage of the safety belt could signal problems with memory. If it isn't that the driver forgets to use the safety belt, but that he or she can't operate it because of physical limitations, there are seat belt extenders that can lengthen the

receptacle and strings or ribbons that can make it easier to pull the belt over the shoulder and torso.

- Difficulty negotiating sharp turns *and intersections.*
  These may reflect problems with seeing or moving, both of which impair safety.

- Hesitating *over right-of-way decisions.*
  This may signal an important problem with cognitive processing speed.

- *Difficulty keeping the car in the proper lane.*
  A driver who straddles lanes, drifts into lanes without realizing it, or changes lanes without signaling could have a vision or movement problem.

GREEN SIGNALS OF RISK

- *Trouble seeing over the steering wheel.*
  The driver's eye level should be between the top of the wheel and the level of the rear-view mirror, approximately 10 inches away from the air bag. Short drivers should use a seat cushion or pillow to achieve the correct position.

- *Difficulty looking back over one's shoulder.*
  Commonly caused by neck stiffness or pain, this can cause real problems. See a driver rehabilitation specialist to find out if getting the car fitted for adaptive mirrors will help, and consult with a healthcare provider to see if there are treatments that can improve flexibility and range of motion.

- *Trouble* physically *moving the steering wheel or looking out mirrors.*
  Again, while relatively minor, these signal problems with movement. Talk to a physician about exercises that may help

the driver maintain the strength and flexibility required to operate a vehicle. Correcting such problems and improving fitness may help avoid more serious problems down the road.

- *Difficulty getting in or out of the vehicle.*
  Improving your total fitness may help improve this. In addition, consider putting something slick, such as a plastic trash bag or a silk scarf over the seat to make it easier to slide in and out of the car.

The Consequences of Ignoring Warning Signs: a Case Study

It seems that you only have to open the newspaper to find an example of an older driver having problems. The consequences of ignoring the kind of risk signals just described range from minor to catastrophic. Unfortunately, catastrophic results do happen. I present the case study below not to sensationalize the issue, but to hammer home the importance of paying attention to even minor warning signs. I reviewed dozens of local and national news accounts, the National Transportation Safety Board reports, and data released from the Santa Monica Police Department to tell the following story, using three perspectives, that of the driver, witnesses, and investigative report.

GEORGE

It was an ordinary day. Despite hip replacements, chronic leg pain, and arthritis, George still got around pretty well with a cane and regularly walked around the neighborhood for exercise. He and his wife lived in a modest, comfortable home and were members of a supportive church. After breakfast he ran a few errands before it got too hot—the week before temperatures had hovered near 100 degrees. He was home for lunch, finished writing a letter, and then drove to the post office. It was a Wednesday afternoon, so traffic wasn't bad. He pulled up to the mailbox in the parking lot, slid across the seat, and dropped the letter into the box. Sliding back to the driver's seat, he put the car back in gear and headed out of the post office parking lot for home. His route home would take him by the popular Santa Monica farmer's market.

THE FARMERS' MARKET

Witnesses were frozen by the sound and motion of it all, likening it to a tornado, tidal wave, and earthquake all hitting at the same time. Bodies and stands were flying like pins in a bowling alley. A crowd rushed the car when it finally came to a stop. They pulled the driver, an elderly man, from the car. Then they lifted the '92 Buick off the woman trapped underneath and disabled the horn, which allowed the other, haunting sounds to take over. Screams of pain and confusion, and calls for help filled the air, as did sirens and, a bit later, the sounds of helicopters coming to transport the injured to hospitals. The Police Chief, James T. Butts, Jr., said it was the single most horrific, devastating scene of tragedy he had ever seen in thirty years of law enforcement. By the end of the week, 10 people were dead and 63 injured. The dead ranged in age from 7 months to 78 years; death came painfully and indiscriminately.

NATIONAL TRANSPORTATION SAFETY BOARD REPORT

On July 16, 2003, about 1:46 p.m. Pacific Daylight Time, a 1992 Buick LeSabre driven by an 86-year old male was westbound on Arizona Avenue, approaching the intersection of Fourth Street, in Santa Monica, Los Angeles County, California. At the same time, a 2003 Mercedes Benz S430 sedan was also westbound on Arizona Avenue and had stopped for pedestrians in a crosswalk. The Buick struck the left rear corner of the Mercedes, continued through the intersection, and drove through a farmers' market, striking pedestrians and vendor displays before coming to rest. The Buick proceeded through the farm-

ers' market for approximately 2 blocks (750 feet) and came to rest near the intersection of Ocean and Arizona Avenues. As a result of the accident, 10 people died and 63 people were injured, some seriously.

The Buick driver stated to police that he tried to stop the car as it went through the market, stepping on the brake, taking his foot off the accelerator, and ultimately trying to put the car's transmission in "park". Police officers were on the scene within one minute and by the end of the afternoon a total of 400 municipal employees (fire, ambulance, police, etc.) responded to the accident. He indicated he might have confused the brake and accelerator pedals.

The results of the National Transportation Safety Board investigation excluded many potential causes of the accident: weather; driver's experience and familiarity with his vehicle and area; alcohol; illicit medications; insufficient sleep or fatigue; pedal placement or vehicle failure. The report concluded that the driver unintentionally accelerated his vehicle. The driver made an error in response execution, inadvertently accelerating when he intended to brake, that resulted in the collision with the Mercedes. The driver failed to detect his error in response execution, thereby inadvertently accelerating his vehicle and propelling it through the Santa Monica farmers' market. The driver most likely reverted to the habitual response of hard braking or "pumping" the brakes as his stress level increased and the vehicle failed to slow, but because his foot was on the accelerator instead of the brake pedal, this response led to increased acceleration. The ineffectiveness of the driver's efforts to stop his vehicle and the realization that he was striking objects in his path very likely increased the already high level of stress affecting him, thereby impeding his ability to quickly detect and correct his earlier error in response execution.

CASE STUDY ANALYSIS

The accident at the Santa Monica Farmers' Market remains nothing less than a personal and national tragedy. On that perfectly ordinary summer day, an intelligent, grandfatherly 86-year-old man was involved in a horrific auto accident. Although no one can ever predict an accident, it turns out that a trained eye *might* have detected enough warning signs to raise concern about his driving fitness. He exhibited several of the warning signs detailed earlier in this chapter. The investigative reports of the accident noted: *vision impairment* (corrected with glasses); *mobility issues* (history of bilateral hip replacement, spinal stenosis, arthritis of such severity that a disabled parking placard was issued; pain in the right thigh, and cane required for walking); and *medication* (prescription and over-the-counter) use. Perhaps most striking of all the warning signs was a *recent history of minor auto accidents* (3 in 10 years). Three weeks after the crash, a cardiologist diagnosed a serious heart problem in George and implanted a dual chamber pacemaker.

Admittedly, hindsight is always 20/20. But in retrospect, it seems that George clearly had enough warning signs to at least raise concerns about his driving fitness. The truth is that predicting future accident risk is not yet an exact science. It is not clear who is responsible for assessment, either. If an older driver cannot or does not heed warning signs, who *should*? A state's department of motor vehicles? The police? Physicians? Family members? Neighbors? Research and vigorous debate about these fundamental policy questions is lacking and yet never more urgently needed. Because you are reading this book, I assume that you have more than a passing interest in the topic. I hope that you will push these questions toward the front burner for decision makers.

Determining Driving Fitness: Ability to See, Think, and Move

This section reviews the main skills and functions needed to safely operate a vehicle. As I've mentioned, in order to drive safely, a person must be able to see, **think,** and **move** well and with ease. If any of these abilities is limited, the driver could be at risk.

SEE

The ability to see is essential to safe driving. For example, we need to be able to read the gauges and dials in the car, see street signs, recover our focus at night, recognize and respond to brake lights, and correctly judge the speed and location of other vehicles around us. Nearly every key task in driving involves detecting, processing, and responding to visual cues. Eye doctors can evaluate *visual acuity,* which is needed to read road signs and to see objects, such as pedestrians or other cars, in the driving path. The useful field of view, or *visual field,* has to do with our peripheral vision, or the ability to see off to the sides without moving our head or eyes. A reduced visual field means that it is harder to see cars and people off to the side. The ability to recover from *glare* changes with age, and older eyes need more time to recover than younger eyes. *Sensitivity to light* is needed to see the taillights of other cars at night. *Depth perception* is the ability to judge the distance between objects, such as oncoming cars, and us.

THINK

Not only do we need to see all the stimuli that surround us, but we also need to make sense of it all by thinking quickly and clearly. Memory, attention, visual attention, and executive function are all high-level skills needed to drive safely. *Divided attention* is used when you are doing two things at once, such as talking to a passenger and navigating a turn. *Selective attention* is the ability to tune out or ignore what is not important in order to focus on what is important. The *speed of thinking* and decision making is critical to driving safety and tends to decrease with aging. Slowed or hesitant responses to situations such as merging or changing lanes are often causes of accidents for older drivers. *Memory* is vital to safe driving. You've got to be able to remember where you are going, the rules of the road, and how to make decisions.

MOVE

In order to drive safely, you need to be able to move without much restriction. Moving in this way requires flexibility and muscle strength. *Flexibility* is the ability to stretch or move a joint or muscle. Being flexible enough to turn to look behind you when backing up or being flexible enough to get in and out of your car are key functions. *Muscle strength* is needed to open the door, change gears, turn the steering wheel, and press the brake and gas pedals.

DRIVING SKILL

A brief mention of general driving proficiency is warranted. You have to know and follow the rules of the road in order to be a safe driver. A lifetime of bad driving habits will catch up with an older driver suddenly faced with problems stemming from health-related changes. A history of aggressive or careless driving does not bode well for future safety. A refresher course should definitely be taken to learn new, safer driving habits.

Assessments of Driver Safety

Below is a description of the range of assessment options available to help you or your loved one to assess driving fitness.

HOME ASSESSMENT

The easiest, most affordable, and comprehensive do-it-yourself home assessment is the Roadwise Review™ program, available from the American Automobile Association (AAA) for a small fee (approximately $15.00). The Roadwise Review™ program is not an assessment of actual driving performance, but it does provide an easy way for you to measure important functional abilities directly related to driving in the comfort of your own home. The program is on CD-ROM and can run on most home personal computers. The only drawback is that it requires access to a computer, and some of us are not experienced or comfortable computer users. If a person's unfamiliarity with computers would lead to results that aren't a valid reflection of his or her abilities, then don't use this program. However, if the older person is familiar with computers, or is interested in learning about them, the Roadwise Review™ gives you an opportunity to generate concrete results about driving fitness that can make your conversations easier.

Driving safely requires complex visual processing, quick and clear thinking, and flexibility and strength. A change or loss in any of these functions (**seeing, thinking, moving**) could endanger you. The Roadwise Review™ program identifies specific impairments that may pose a risk in many common driving situations and provides a good general discussion of driving fitness. Eight areas are reviewed:

1. *Leg strength and general mobility:* you need these functions to accelerate and brake under regular conditions and to respond quickly in emergencies.

2. *Head/neck flexibility:* this allows you to check blind spots when you back up, change lanes, and merge into traffic.

3. *High-contrast visual acuity:* this helps you detect pavement markings, read road signs, and spot hazards in or near the road.

4. *Low-contrast visual acuity:* this enables you to maintain lane position and drive safely in rain, dusk, haze, and fog.

5. *Working memory:* this allows you to follow directions, remember traffic rules and regulations, and make good decisions as you drive.

6. *Visualizing missing information:* this enables you to recognize and anticipate a threat or hazard even when part of it is hidden from view.

7. *Visual search:* this enables you to scan the driving environment and recognize traffic signs, signals, navigational landmarks, and hazards.

8. *Visual information processing speed:* this allows you to pay attention to what is in front of you while also detecting threats at the edge of your field of view.

This assessment requires two people, the driver and a helper. It also requires a stable, straight-back chair that does not roll, tilt, or swivel; a measured 10-foot path near the computer; and about an hour to complete. The results are completely private and available for your review after completing the program. I recommend it as an excellent first step in determining your driving fitness.

ASSESSMENT BY A HEALTHCARE PROVIDER

If an in-home assessment suggests a problem, the next step would be to consult with the older person's physician or another healthcare provider in order to do a more thorough evaluation. This typically will not involve an actual road test, which is the final and most definitive level of assessment.

Recognizing the growing importance of evaluating driving ability among older adults, the American Medical Association created an assessment guideline for physicians called the Assessment of Driving-Related Skills (ADReS). This is a set of brief tests, conducted in a doctor's office, which measures the three key functions for safe driving (vision, cognition, and motor function). Some physicians may use other systems or they may have developed their own strategies for assessing function. If your physician is not familiar with the ADReS, it can be freely accessed via the internet from the professional resources section (Public Health: Geriatric Health) of the AMA Web site (www.ama-assn.org or via the National Highway Transportation Safety Administration at www.nhtsa.dot.gov/people/injury/olddrive/OlderDriversBook). Here's a brief overview of the ADReS evaluation and what you or a loved one can expect.

ADReS Vision Exams

Aspects of vision that are important for safe driving can be assessed by most primary care physicians. Far *visual acuity* is assessed using the standard Snellen E Chart. With the chart hung at the proper distance the patient reads the smallest line of text possible. The visual acuity score is based on the lowest full-row read. One's field of view is measured by what is called confrontational testing. The examiner sits or stands 3 feet in front of the patient, at the patient's eye level. The patient is asked to close his or her right eye, while the examiner closes his or her left eye. Each fixes on the other's nose. The examiner then holds up a random number of fingers in each of four quadrants and asks the patient to state the number of fingers. The process is repeated for each eye.

ADReS Cognitive Exams

General *cognitive function* is measured with the Trail-Making Test (Part B), in which the person is asked to draw a line between small circles on a page in a specified order.

Research indicates that poor performance on the test is associated with poor driving performance. Another simple evaluation of memory, visual perception, and executive skills is the Clock Drawing Test. In this test the examiner gives the patient a piece of paper and a pencil and asks him/her to draw a clock, including the face and numbers, and to indicate the time as specified.

ADReS Motor Function Exams

The *Rapid Pace Walk* is used to measure lower limb strength, endurance, range of motion, and balance. A 10-foot path is marked and the patient is asked to walk the path, turn around, and walk back to the starting point as quickly as possible. The *Manual Test of Range of Motion* and *Manual Test of Motor Strength* are simple subjective tests of resistance to an examiner's pressing or of measurements of the range of motion of the head or extremities.

Assessment by a Driving Rehabilitation Specialist

An assessment by a driving rehabilitation specialist or geriatric driving clinic is the most comprehensive test of driving fitness, but it's also the most time-consuming and expensive. An assessment at a program like the DriveWise program at Beth Israel Deaconess Medical Center in Boston, Massachusetts, takes two patient visits to complete. Visit One, the actual multidisciplinary assessment, takes four hours and involves a social worker, a neuropsychologist, a nurse, an occupational therapist, and a certified driving rehabilitation specialist. First, an assessment conducted by a social worker determines driving needs and driving history, driving-related knowledge, license status, and a complete medical and medication history. Then a neuropsychological evaluation is done to assess cognitive status, followed by an evaluation with an occupational therapist to examine reflexes, vision, and mental status. Finally, an actual road test assessment is conducted by a certified driving rehabilitation specialist. In Visit Two about two weeks later, the findings are reviewed with the driver and family.

Driving assessment clinics are often based in academic medical centers (teaching hospitals) or at outpatient rehabilitation clinics. This type of assessment tends to be the most expensive (around $400 or so) and is not yet covered by health insurance. However, many older drivers and family members have reported that the peace of mind afforded by such a comprehensive assessment is worth every penny.

Medical Conditions That Increase Driving Risk

Many of us have been driving so long that it feels just about automatic—as if we could drive a familiar route with our eyes closed. It's easy to forget how complicated a task driving really is. But safe driving requires the quick and continuous processing of incoming sensory information, the coordination of muscles and quick reflexes, and a host of mental processes such as accessing and updating long-term memories. As I noted in the previous chapter, this boils down to an ability to **see, think,** and **move** well enough to drive safely.

Unfortunately, many medical conditions can impair these three key skills—and the incidence of such conditions increases with age. Sometimes the effects of a medical problem are obvious and occur suddenly—injury to an eye, for example, or a broken hip. But many chronic conditions develop gradually, and their effects on driving ability are more difficult to detect. In addition, the *treatments* for some conditions can impair driving as much as—or more than—the conditions themselves. For example, opioid medications that can work such wonders to relieve intense, chronic pain can also impair thinking ability and alertness.

This chapter explores the most common medical conditions that biomedical research has shown can affect driving ability. I briefly describe each condition, explain why or how the condition or its treatment may affect driving, and then, when it's appropriate, I give you some advice about how to manage the condition so that you or a loved one can continue driving safely.

Before I begin, however, I'd like you to note the following:

Not every condition or disease that could potentially affect driving performance is described in this chapter. I have only included those conditions identified through empirical research or noted in national clinical practice guidelines. Because evidence is lacking on so many common illnesses and events, let me apologize in advance if the condition you are interested in is not discussed. For example, you'll notice that there's no information about cancer, even though it's extremely common in older adults and some cancers (or their treatment) certainly can adversely affect driving. My own current research explores whether a link exists between breast cancer and driving safety in older women. Since more than 30% of women treated for breast cancer may report an upper body symptom (such as pain, swelling, or infection) at one year post treatment, it seems reasonable to suspect a potential association with driving problems. However, the research results will not be available for several years. These frustrating gaps in the biomedical literature highlight the important need for public and private investments in geriatric research.

Not every person with one of the conditions noted in this chapter will have problems with driving performance. Having a medical condition is simply a signal or warning sign that there *could be* a safe-driving issue. They are described here to alert you to a possible risk. Many people, however, even those with multiple chronic conditions, can drive safely with proper treatment and/or the use of assistive technologies (described in Chapter 8).

This chapter provides general information; it does not offer medical advice. Always talk to a healthcare provider about a medical condition and how it may, or may not, affect your driving. Be aware that not all physicians are comfortable or trained to discuss driving fitness issues, so don't be afraid to ask your healthcare providers if they are. If you're not satisfied with answers you get, don't hesitate to seek a second opinion.

―――――――――――DISORDERS OF VISION―――――――――――

Janet had perfect 20/20 vision until she turned 42. Then, like many people in their 40s, she needed to wear eyeglasses in order to crochet or read. At first, she didn't need glasses to drive, but by her mid-50s she did. About 10 years after that, when she was 67, Janet was driving back to Minneapolis from Minnesota's north shore at dusk. She was wearing her glasses, but she noticed that everything "looked brown" and it was hard for her to judge distances. Not long after that, she was driving home from the movies one night and couldn't see well enough to turn corners properly. Alarmed, she went to her eye doctor. She was told she had cataracts that didn't require surgery but that could affect her driving ability.

Janet had always been a safe and cautious driver, and she decided not to drive at night anymore. She also decided to do her best to avoid driving during bad weather or when the light was dim even during the day. Now 70, she continues to follow these rules she has set for herself. As she put it, she doesn't have the ability to see the "whole picture" when she is driving at night or in low-light conditions. Janet recognized that her vision problems put her at risk during night driving, so she modified her behavior to reduce the risk to herself and others.

Of the five senses, vision is by far the most important for all drivers, regardless of age. In fact, about 90 percent of the information needed to drive safely relates to the ability to see clearly. Visual impairment is a common problem faced by older adults. Sometimes the impairment is simply the result of age-related physiological changes. You may find it helpful to refer to this diagram of eye anatomy from The National Eye Institute, of the National Institutes of Health.

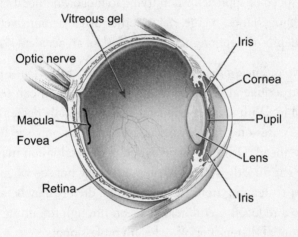

The most common age-related changes are the reduced clarity of the cornea, lens, and interior fluids of the eyes. These changes can cut the amount of light reaching the back of the eye of a 60-year-old by two-thirds compared to the average 20-year-old. In addition, the lens of the eye becomes stiffer with age, which impairs focusing on near objects. These common age-related changes may affect driving performance in a variety of ways:

• *Reduced dynamic visual acuity*: Dynamic visual acuity is the ability to see a moving object, especially when there isn't much light—such as at dawn or dusk, when the weather is foggy, or when the skies are overcast. With age, our eyes tend to lose their dynamic visual acuity, and it becomes harder to see well when there isn't much light.

• *Reduced depth perception*: Depth perception is the ability to determine the distance between us and an object or the *changing* distances between two moving objects. Older drivers tend to use *only* the distance of an approaching vehicle rather than distance *and* its speed of approach when trying to judge whether it's safe to turn, change lanes, merge, or use other driving maneuvers. Reduced depth perception increases the risk of an accident.

• *Narrowed field of view or narrowed peripheral vision*: Field of view, or peripheral vision, is the total area that you can see and respond to. With aging, peripheral vision gradually decreases. In extreme cases one has "tunnel vision" and can only see what is directly ahead. Drivers with impaired peripheral vision may only see the car directly in front of them and may not see when a pedestrian is stepping from the curb. Some drivers may be able to adapt to a reduced useful field of vision through retraining by an occupational therapist or other health professional.

• *Reduced contrast sensitivity*: Contrast sensitivity is the capacity to sharply see the difference between two similarly colored objects. Changes in the transparency of the lens in the eye can change the perception of color and background. When driving, the inability to see the difference in contrast affects distance judgment. Drivers may have difficulty in determining distance to an object, resulting in tailgating or hitting a curb.

• *Reduced perceptual reaction time*: Perceptual reaction time is the speed with which the driver can process visual information. As we age, not only does this reaction time slow down, but the overall responsiveness of the brain to what the eye senses erodes.

In addition to these normal changes associated with aging, many specific conditions can further impair vision and, thus, the ability to drive safely. These are described below.

MACULAR DEGENERATION

The macula is the part of the retina that allows you to see fine detail. The retina is the light-sensitive tissue lining the back of the eye. Degeneration of the macula leads to a loss or significant blurring of one's central vision. I find a bull's-eye analogy helpful in understanding this condition. If you think of your vision as a bull's-eye, the disease first takes the center circle, or the bull's-eye (central vision), but the outside rings (peripheral vision) remain. As the disease worsens, the loss of central vision expands.

A sign of early-stage macular degeneration is that straight lines or objects appear warped or slanted. If you suspect a problem, you should have your vision checked immediately, since new medications are being developed that may slow the progression of macular degeneration. Many assistive technologies allow people with macular degeneration to continue to read, work on computers, live independently, and even drive safely.

CATARACTS

A cataract is a clouding of the lens in one or both eyes which blurs vision, diminishes color perception, and reduces the overall amount of light entering the eye. Cataracts are so common that by age 80, more than half of all Americans either have a cataract or have had cataract surgery.

The symptoms of a cataract are cloudy or blurry vision, faded colors, poor night vision, and problems with glare. Headlights, lamps, or sunlight may appear too bright; a halo may appear around lights. Another symptom is double vision or multiple images in one eye. (Ironically, this symptom may clear as the cataract gets larger.) Frequent prescription changes in your eyeglasses or contact lenses may be caused by a growing cataract.

GLAUCOMA

Glaucoma is a group of diseases characterized by excessive pressure within the eye, which damages the optic nerve and results in vision loss or blindness. Although damage caused by glaucoma cannot be reversed, early detection and treatment can halt the process and preserve sight.

Glaucoma typically causes no symptoms or pain at first and vision remains normal. But if it remains untreated, people slowly lose their peripheral vision until they view the world as if through a tube. Eventually all vision is lost. The driving-related danger is that a person may have early-stage glaucoma and a related reduction in peripheral vision without knowing it.

DIABETIC RETINOPATHY

Diabetic retinopathy is a complication of diabetes and a leading cause of blindness. It occurs when diabetes damages the tiny blood vessels inside the retina. Like glaucoma, diabetic retinopathy often has no early warning signs.

Blood vessels damaged from diabetic retinopathy can cause vision loss in two ways:

• Fragile blood vessels can leak blood into the center of the eye, blurring vision or causing spots or "floaters" to appear in one's field of view.

• Fluid can leak into the center of the macula, the part of the eye where sharp, straight-ahead vision occurs. The fluid makes the macula swell, blurring vision.

<u>MY ADVICE</u>

Problems with vision don't automatically mean you need to stop driving. Sometimes relatively simple accommodations can be made for declining function. For instance, many visual disorders cause people to need more light than normal to see well. In that case, avoid driving at night or during storms, when light is limited. Vision disorders can also make drivers especially sensitive to light or have difficulty with glare. Again, these people should avoid driving at night to avoid the glare of headlights or in low-light conditions.

Some vision problems can be corrected, such as with lens replacements for cataracts or laser surgery to correct acuity problems. If a condition such as diabetes or glaucoma is being actively managed, further vision loss can be slowed or avoided.

Good vision is so important to safe driving that you must do everything you can to keep your eyes in good shape and correct any problems, if possible. I suggest that you get your eyes examined at least once a year so that any problems are caught early before they do significant damage. Try to see the same eye specialist each year so that she or he can become familiar with your status. Remember to wear your glasses if you have a prescription, and use proper lighting to read. When driving, be aware of the difficulties of shifting quickly from light to dark areas (and vice versa), such as when you enter or exit a tunnel. If you have any doubts about your own vision or that of a loved one, talk to a vision specialist; he or she can tell you whether or not it is safe to drive with your condition.

Because we could all be helped by having an extra mirror or two, or something to help deal with glare, consider establishing a connection with a low vision specialist in your area. Such specialists often know where to obtain and how to use assistive technologies that can help to maintain your driving and overall independence. Many senior and community organizations and agencies offer information about low vision counseling, training, and other special services for people with visual impairments. A school of medicine or optometry may be an excellent resource for low vision services.

───────DISORDERS OF THOUGHT: DEMENTIA───────

The locked door into the dementia care unit buzzed open, and I made my way back to my father's room. At only 76, he was suffering from advanced-stage dementia and was no longer able to walk, talk, dress, feed himself, or take himself to the toilet. It was hard now to remember what the earliest signs of his brain disorder were. Not remembering things we had just talked about? Getting lost driving to the lake even though we had gone there every summer? Those first symptoms had occurred nearly ten years ago, and he had continued to drive for years after that. Thankfully, once diagnosed, his doctor ordered his complete driving retirement because of the side effects of the medication prescribed to manage the behavioral symptoms. The explanation allowed my father to save face—he didn't have to stop driving because he was impaired, but because of this essential medication.

Dementia causes an inevitable decline in cognitive functioning. Symptoms include memory loss and at least one other type of cognitive deficit such as difficulty with speech, decision-making, or social functioning. Dementia is *not* a normal part of aging. All forms of dementia, including Alzheimer's disease, can impair the ability to drive safely by eroding memory, attention span, judgment, vision, and even the ability to recognize that a problem exists in the first place.

With dementia, it is not a question of *if* a person must stop driving, but *when*. There is no wriggle room with this condition. Until a cure is discovered, or at least until better treatments are developed, driving cessation is unavoidable. Early in the disease, if impairment is minimal, limited driving may still be permissible.

However, the progression of the disease can be so subtle that it can be hard for a driver or loved one to know precisely when to stop driving. Close communication with your healthcare provider is essential. Research in this area has only recently begun, and there is some debate among experts about whether immediate driving cessation is indicated for dementia. I tend to think stopping sooner, rather than later, is the best decision.

<u>MY ADVICE</u>

Since dementia is progressive, it makes sense to talk about driving retirement (cessation) as soon as a diagnosis is made—even if driving is not, at the moment, limited. Creating a plan in advance for a gradual transition to driving cessation is a key step. If possible, it's best to reach an understanding and agree on a plan before the disease is too far advanced.

————TRANSIENT ISCHEMIC ATTACKS AND STROKE————

Debbie hung up the phone in disbelief. After living in a lovely retirement community in Arizona for nearly six years, her mother Noreen and stepfather Fred had "decided to pack it all up and to hit the road." Within weeks, they sold their home and were driving a shiny, new recreation vehicle loaded with every conceivable amenity.

Eighteen months later, the thrill wasn't gone. In fact, Fred and Noreen said they'd never felt so happy and alive. They loved seeing the country up close and having the freedom to go wherever, whenever, they chose. They cherished the many new friends and the active social life of the RV parks.

Then, on a crisp autumn afternoon as Fred was slowing down to exit a highway, the vision in his right eye suddenly constricted. It seemed as though he were entering a dark tunnel. His head was throbbing and he felt a tingling weakness in his right arm and leg. Somehow he managed to stop the RV safely right there on the exit ramp. Noreen grabbed the cell phone and dialed 911. Twenty minutes later Fred was in a hospital undergoing tests to figure out what had happened.

Fred was relatively lucky. Not only did he avoid an accident, but his problem was much less serious than the stroke he was afraid he had suffered. In fact, one of the blood vessels feeding part of Fred's brain had gone into spasm, which temporarily had cut off oxygen and produced the stroke-like symptoms. He would come to learn that such spasms are called transient ischemic attacks.

After Fred recovered from his attack, he and Noreen took a hard look at their options. They decided that they'd rather reduce their risk of an accident than continue their nomadic lifestyle. They sold their RV, settled down, established relationships with good healthcare providers, and feel good about their decision.

Transient Ischemic Attacks

Transient ischemic attacks, or TIAs, temporarily cut off oxygen to part of the brain. This can produce dizziness, blurred vision, pain or tingling in the head or limbs, loss of muscle control, or fainting. Fortunately TIAs usually resolve themselves and leave no noticeable symptoms or long-term deficits. However, having a TIA is a warning signal that the person is at risk for a more serious and debilitating stroke. In a given year, approximately 50,000 Americans have a TIA; about one-third of them will have an acute stroke at some point in the future.

Stroke

A stroke can cause many symptoms that impair driving, including problems with coordination, hearing, judgment, motor skills, and thinking. As with all medical conditions, a medical assessment made by a doctor is essential to determine whether or not someone should drive. In addition to a medical diagnosis, a driver's road test can help assess driver competence and safety after a stroke.

<u>*MY ADVICE*</u>

When a stroke occurs, it can affect the skills necessary for independent driving. However, a majority of stroke survivors can return to independent driving. Adaptive equipment is available to counteract physical problems. For example, a spinner knob can be attached to the steering wheel to allow controlled steering with the use of one hand. A left-foot gas pedal can be installed if a driver is unable to use the right foot. Chapter 8 describes a number of these assistive devices. Training by a driving rehabilitation specialist is essential before such equipment can be used safely.

Other Medical Conditions

CARDIOVASCULAR DISEASE

Cardiovascular disease refers to any disorder in your heart or blood vessels such as heart attacks, angina, valve problems, or heart rhythm problems. Cardiovascular disease includes coronary heart disease, myocardial infarction, angina pectoris, and sudden cardiac death. The connection between cardiovascular diseases and driving is that these conditions increase the chance that the driver will lose consciousness behind the wheel. In addition, medications used to treat these conditions can impair alertness or motor function.

<u>*MY ADVICE*</u>

See your cardiologist or primary care physician regularly to manage any cardiovascular condition you or a loved one might have. If prescription or over-the-counter medications are taken, be sure to keep healthcare providers informed about *all* of the drugs being taken to avoid any dangerous interactions. If appropriate, be diligent in your cardiac rehabilitation program: improving your cardiac fitness is likely to yield benefits to your overall driving fitness as well.

CHRONIC OBSTRUCTIVE PULMONARY DISEASE

Chronic obstructive pulmonary disease (COPD) is caused by the partial blockage of the airways in the lungs, making it difficult to breathe. Cigarette smoking is the most common cause of COPD. Breathing in other kinds of lung irritants, like pollution, dust, or chemicals over a long period of time may also cause or contribute to COPD. COPD develops slowly, and it may be many years before there are noticeable symptoms such as shortness of breath. Most of the time, COPD is diagnosed in middle-aged or older people. Feeling short of breath may be distracting while driving or may impair thinking.

MY ADVICE

Since there is no known cure for COPD, treatment is usually aimed at relieving symptoms and improving quality of life. People with COPD may be able to drive for a while, but eventually breathing becomes so labored that driving is no longer possible. Start talking about driving as soon as COPD is diagnosed. Prepare for when driving will not be possible.

DIABETES

Almost 20 million American adults have diabetes, and the incidence of this disease increases dramatically with age and obesity. Diabetes makes it difficult for the body to control the levels of sugar in the blood. Excessive blood sugar levels cause a wide range of problems in addition to the retinopathy mentioned earlier. The most critical complication related to driving is the possibility of an episode of very low blood sugar, called a hypoglycemic attack. Such attacks can cause dizziness or fainting, both of which would obviously be dangerous while driving. People having an active episode of either low or high blood sugar should not drive. Also, they shouldn't drive if they have repeated hypoglycemic or hyperglycemic attacks. Symptoms of hypoglycemia include: hunger, nervousness and shakiness, perspiration, dizziness or light-headedness, sleepiness, confusion, difficulty speaking, and feeling anxious or weak. The signs and symptoms of hyperglycemia include: high blood glucose, high levels of sugar in the urine, frequent urination, and increased thirst. It's very important to treat hyperglycemia as soon as you detect it because of the risk of diabetic coma (ketoacidosis).

MY ADVICE

Drivers who have diabetes should work with their doctor to manage the disease and to control symptoms. In many cases, if a driver's symptoms are under control, diabetes will not increase driving risk. However, only a doctor can determine whether these symptoms are under control.

ARTHRITIS

What most people call arthritis is actually a collection of more than 100 different types of conditions that cause pain in the joints and connective tissue throughout the body. The key symptoms are joint pain, stiffness, swelling, and redness. Loss of joint mobility may result in diminished ability to reach, grasp, manipulate, and release objects, such as the steering wheel or gear shift. Strength, endurance, and range of motion difficulties may require that adaptive devices be installed in a car, such as extra mirrors, key holders, extended gear shift levers, power windows, and door locks. As I mentioned earlier, Chapter 8 describes a number of assistive devices that may help.

MY ADVICE

Talk to your doctor about your symptoms. Discuss ways to increase your range of motion and control your pain without impairing your ability to drive. Starting an exercise program with the advice of your physician can help. Often, a healthcare provider will refer you to a physical and occupational therapist who can work to improve your range of motion and function and who will have catalogs of assistive devices. For instance, if you have a permanent decreased range of motion of your neck, your car may be fitted with mirrors to reduce blind spots.

PARKINSON'S DISEASE

Parkinson's disease is a movement disorder that affects about 1.5 million Americans, most of whom are older than 65. The major features of Parkinson's disease are impaired movement, tremor, and uncontrolled hand motions. The disease is also associated with a low-volume voice, diminished facial expression, and gait problems. All of these clinical features may affect physical and mental abilities, which in turn can reduce driving ability. Parkinson's disease is progressive, which means that motor and cognitive impairments will inevitably worsen over time.

MY ADVICE

People with Parkinson's disease should be monitored by their primary care physician regularly (at least every 6 to 12 months), and during these ongoing checkups, driving safety should be openly discussed. Eventually, the effects of Parkinson's disease will become so strong that a person suffering from it will no longer be able to drive safely.

DEPRESSION

Some people think that depression is a normal part of the aging process, but it isn't. Depression is a real, serious medical condition. It often occurs in combination with other serious illnesses such as heart disease, stroke, diabetes, cancer, and Parkinson's disease. It should be treated in conjunction with any other condition that a person has. Depression can cause lethargy, drowsiness, or inattentiveness to one's surroundings. It can also make a person physically slow. A depressed person can lose the ability to concentrate or to become agitated. Depression can also cause bleak or suicidal thoughts. People who are suicidal or who are experiencing severe symptoms of depression or any mental illness should never drive.

MY ADVICE

Drivers who have been diagnosed with depression should work with their doctor to manage the disease and to control symptoms. In most cases, if a driver's symptoms are under control, depression will not increase driving risk. However, only you and your doctor can determine whether these symptoms are under control. Also, some medications used to treat depression and other psychiatric illnesses can impair driving ability. (See Chapter 3 for more on medications and driving safety.)

ANXIETY

Of the various types of anxiety disorders, panic attacks are the type most likely to interfere with driving. A person having a panic attack can feel like they're suffocating, they can be agitated and inattentive, or they can simply be unable to concentrate on anything except their racing heartbeat, sweaty palms, and other uncomfortable symptoms. Panic attacks can be triggered by situations commonly experienced while driving, such as cross-ing bridges, being stuck in traffic, driving near steep drop-offs, or getting lost.

MY ADVICE

Because anxiety disorders usually get worse if untreated and tend to respond very well to treatment, this is something you don't want to ignore. Be sure to seek medical attention for anxiety from a trained professional. Your primary care provider should be able to recommend one. The treatment is likely to include psychotherapy (such as talking to a counselor skilled in cognitive-behavioral therapy or behavioral therapy) and medication. Be aware, however, that nearly all medications prescribed for anxiety can impair driving fitness.

The key with any medical condition, whether your own or that of a loved one, is clear communication, an honest, ongoing relationship with a healthcare provider, and obtaining and maintaining effective treatment. Doing so will not only preserve your driving ability, but will likely improve your total quality of life.

CHAPTER 3

Driving and Drugs:

Prescription and Over-the-Counter Medications, Vitamins, and Herbal Supplements

Medicine today is full of great promise as well as new challenges. The dizzying rate at which new medications are being discovered is nothing less than amazing. Diseases and conditions that in the past tended to remain unmentioned, undiagnosed, and untreated (such as overactive bladder or erectile dysfunction) now have an array of available remedies. Medications have unquestionably improved both longevity and quality of life. But these tools for health must be used carefully: errors in prescribing, filling, consuming, or combining medications can be hazardous or even fatal. And even when medications are prescribed and taken correctly, they can impair driving ability.

Adults age 65 and older consume more prescription and over-the-counter medication than people in any other age group. A recent national survey of the noninstitutionalized (that is, those *not* living in a nursing home, hospital, or other care facility) adult U.S. population found that more than 90% of people 65 or older use at least one medication per week. Approximately one half (46%) take five or more prescription medications, and 12% take 10 or more different medications per week. Many older adults have several different conditions that need to be treated by multiple medications. But it's not uncommon for two or more different medications to be used to treat a *single* condition. This is especially true of conditions that are particularly common among older adults such as high blood pressure, heart failure, diabetes, and Alzheimer's disease.

Many prescription and nonprescription drugs and supplements can affect driving ability, yet these effects are often overlooked—both by patients and their physicians. It's particularly important to be aware of these medication-related issues because sometimes a problem with driving is caused solely by a medication. In such cases, a change in medication may fix the problem.

Unfortunately research on older drivers and medication safety is sparse. The information in this chapter is based on published medical studies and data provided by the American Medical Association, the National Institutes of Health, the Food and Drug Administration, and other recognized medical and scientific authorities. The chapter provides an overview of medication safety and then presents information about the most common classes of drugs that can impair driving ability. I also take a look at vitamins and herbal supplements because, surprisingly, even these can affect driving.

It is important to note that **not every medication that could possibly affect driving performance is described here. Further, this chapter provides general information, not medical advice. To learn more about a particular medication, please check with your pharmacist or healthcare professional.** At the end of this chapter I include questions to ask your pharmacist or doctor to enhance the safety of any medications you or a loved one may be taking. Appendix 3 includes the names and addresses of resources that can provide you with more detailed information.

Medication Safety: An Overview

We take medications to fix a problem or to improve our health. However, many drugs can cause side effects that can compromise our ability to drive safety. If you are taking two or more medications, they can also interact with each other to create different side effects that can pose a risk to your driving safety. Although vitamins and herbal supplements are not considered medications by most, they can affect your physical and mental skills, and they can also interact dangerously with each other or with medications. You should tell your doctor about **all** of the medications and supplements that you are taking every time you see him or her.

Medications are usually divided into one of two groups: prescription medications and over-the-counter (OTC) drugs. Prescription medications are those drugs that require a doctor's prescription to buy and are used to treat specific diseases and symptoms. Over-the-counter drugs are those that you can buy without a prescription. Common OTC drugs include pain relievers such as Tylenol® and Advil®, cold and allergy medications such as Sudafed® and Claritin-D®, and antacids such as Tums® and Prilosec OTC®. Over-the-counter drugs also include generic or store-brand versions of name-brand drugs. Vitamins and nutritional supplements are not considered medications, but they can have some of the same positive and negative effects on us that medications do.

The effects of medications vary from person to person and can be based on the dosage or amount of medication that you take, your medical condition, and other drugs that you are taking. Read the labels on all the drugs and supplements you are taking and heed any warnings about drug interactions. If a label on one drug says that another drug is "contraindicated," that means that you should not take both drugs. Talk to your doctor or pharmacist if you have any questions about drug interactions.

The effects of a medication also depend on your age. As we get older, changes occur in our bodies that alter how drugs affect us. In general, the older we get, the longer it takes the liver to break down (metabolize) a drug, and the longer that drug will stay in our bodies. Also, as we age, we may need less than the recommended adult dosage for some medications. Talk to your doctor about dosage amounts and your age and health.

The effects of some drugs can also depend on how long you've been taking it. When you start taking a medication, side effects can be at their worst. Often, however, your body adjusts to the medication and side effects lessen. This means you or a loved one should be particularly careful about driving during the initial stages of taking any medication until you know exactly how it will affect you. Conversely, some medications—Valium, for example—build up in your body over time. Also, changes in your physical or mental condition can affect how you react to a medication, even if you've been taking the medication a long time. If you notice any changes in how a drug seems to be affecting you, contact your doctor or healthcare professional.

It's always good practice to get your prescriptions and over-the-counter medications at the same pharmacy. Try to get to know the pharmacist(s); they are professionals who can help you manage your medications safely. One advantage of using one pharmacy is that the staff will have a record of your medications, be aware of your medication history, and can easily spot potentially hazardous drug combinations. The technology available now means that even rare, but dangerous, drug interactions can be spotted in the pharmacy's computerized records.

You should also read and heed the warning labels on prescription and OTC medications and on supplements. I know this isn't always easy—the labels and inserts are often printed in very small type and are not written in everyday language. But usually the really important information is printed in **boldface,** which makes it easier to spot. Be especially careful if the label says the medication could cause drowsiness or agitation, or if it warns against operating a vehicle while taking the drug. Do not drive until you know how these medications affect you. Some medications will have short-acting side effects such as nausea that will last for a couple of hours after you take a dose. If you know that you will experience such side effects, you should plan your driving schedule accordingly.

Alcohol

Alcohol is the most commonly used drug in our society. Alcohol was involved in about 40% of the fatal motor vehicle accidents in the U.S. in 2004. The death toll is enormous, and yet the risk posed by drinking and driving is still widely ignored or not understood. The problem is simple: the amount of alcohol in even a single beer, glass of wine, or shot of hard liquor impairs **seeing, thinking,** and **moving,** the three key skills required for safe driving. The impact on thinking is crucial because it causes people to underestimate the degree of their own impairment. Drivers arrested for drunk driving often claim that they felt perfectly safe to drive. This impact on self-judgment paired with the muscle incoordination, vision disturbances, and slowed reaction times caused by alcohol combine to make alcohol our biggest drug-related driving hazard.

The negative effects of alcohol can be particularly acute for older drivers—though as I noted earlier in the Introduction, older drivers as a class actually are much *less* likely to drive under the influence than younger drivers. Older adults metabolize alcohol more slowly, meaning that they will remain intoxicated longer than a younger person after ingesting a given amount of alcohol. Age-related changes in body composition (increase in fat, decrease in water) combine to make the concentration of alcohol greater. Thus, for people who used to enjoy two cocktails when they were in their 40s, they find that they can't handle that amount in their 60s or 70s. Also, older adults are more likely to be taking a prescription or OTC medication—such as many cough remedies, sleeping pills, or anti-anxiety medications—that enhances the sedating effects of alcohol. All of this makes it imperative to heed the commonsense admonition: if you drink, don't drive. Period.

Anticholinergics

Anticholinergics block the effects of acetylcholine, a natural body chemical that helps transmit signals between nerve cells. Anticholinergics are common in many prescription and OTC medications, including those used to treat depression, allergies, nausea, Parkinson's disease, and serious mental illnesses. The side effects of anticholinergics can impair driving many ways since they can cause

- blurred vision

- drowsiness or sedation

- confusion

- tremors

- impaired memory

- lack of coordination

Ask your doctor or pharmacist if any of the prescription *or* OTC medications you're using contains an anticholinergic compound and, if so, be extremely cautious about driving. Also, never combine the medication with alcohol.

Anticonvulsants

Anticonvulsants are generally prescribed for controlling seizures and for treating epilepsy. They are also sometimes prescribed for the treatment of bipolar disorder, mania, or anxiety, and sometimes for other reasons such as for controlling migraine headaches or other kinds of pain. Some commonly prescribed anticonvulsants are Depakene® (valproic acid), Depakote® (divalproex), Dilantin® (phenytoin), Lamictal® (lamotrigine), Tegretol® (carbamazepine), and Topamax® (topiramate).

Anticonvulsants can cause blurred vision, dizziness, tremors, and limitation of motor skills and coordination. You or a loved one shouldn't drive when you first start taking anticonvulsants, during any period when you change the amount you are taking, or during the period when you gradually stop taking them. During these times, the risk of seizure is high, which makes it unsafe to drive. Anticonvulsants can still be impairing once you're on a steady dose, so you should be cautious about driving whenever you're taking such drugs and ask your doctor for his or her advice about driving.

Anticonvulsants are often prescribed in conjunction with other medications, those that treat bipolar disorder (called antipsychotics) or anxiety (called anxiolytics). When taken in combination with these other drugs, anticonvulsants have much stronger impairing effects, especially on motor skills. You shouldn't drive if you are taking a combination of anticonvulsants and antipsychotics or of anticonvulsants and anxiolytics.

Antidepressants

Although depression itself is a risk factor for unsafe driving, the medications used to *treat* depression can also impair driving ability. Several classes of antidepressants exist and some have more sedating or impairing side effects than others. But any antidepressant, particularly during the first weeks of administration, can cause side effects in some people that can affect driving, such as

- drowsiness

- lightheadedness or dizziness

- anxiety

- restlessness

- inattentiveness

- tremors

If you have begun a course of antidepressants, you should refrain from driving until you determine what, if any, side effects you may experience. It usually takes 4 to 6 weeks for an antidepressant to take effect fully and it's during this time that side effects are usually strongest. If side effects are minimal or if they lessen with time, you can drive safely.

Depression can strike at any age, but tends to be dramatically underdiagnosed in older adults. For example, depression sometimes

accompanies serious illness or diseases such as cancer, heart attack, or chronic pain and is never detected or treated. In addition,
depression can sometimes be a complication of the normal griev-
ing process involved with losing a loved one, retiring, or coping
with limitations on one's independence. The good news is that current treatments for depression—both with medications and "talk"
therapy—can be very effective. But anybody using an antidepressant, particularly in the early phases, should be aware of the possible adverse effects on their driving.

Antiemetics

Antiemetics treat nausea, vomiting, dizziness, or diarrhea
caused by diseases, conditions, or certain medical treatments such
as chemotherapy, radiation therapy, or surgery. Antiemetics can
compromise driving performance because they can cause drowsiness, blurred vision, headache, confusion, and lack of coordination.
Often, a person can be seriously impaired by these drugs without
being aware of it. People taking antiemetics should be very cautious
about driving.

Antihistamines

Antihistamines are found in many medications for allergies,
colds, and flu. Some antihistamines are also prescribed for other
reasons, such as to treat motion sickness, Parkinson's disease, or
sleeplessness. Antihistamines can impair safe driving because they
can cause drowsiness and muscle incoordination. They can also
affect your ability to think clearly.

Some antihistamines have a strong sedating effect on people,
even when taken in normal doses. These sedating antihistamines
include chlorpheniramine (also known as Chlor-Trimeton®, among

other brands) and diphenhydramine. Diphenhydramine is most commonly known by the brand name Benadryl®, but it is also an ingredient in many over-the-counter sleep aids, such as Nytol®, Unisom®, and Excedrin P.M.®. People taking these kinds of antihistamines shouldn't drive, even if they don't feel sleepy.

Most nonsedating antihistamines such as fexofenadine (Allegra®) and loratadine (Claritin®) will not impair driving. However, some of them *can* be a problem, especially if they are taken at doses that are higher than recommended. And at least one nonsedating antihistamine—cetirizine (Zyrtec®)—can cause impairments in some people even if taken in normal doses. Be cautious because when a problem is found with one drug in a class, in time problems are usually found with other similar drugs. So people taking these nonsedating antihistamines should use caution when determining whether or not to drive.

Antihypertensives

Antihypertensive drugs treat high blood pressure (hypertension). More than 65 million American adults have some degree of hypertension—that's about one in three. Some people with hypertension experience dizziness, heart palpitations, fainting, or headache. Hypertension can also lead to damage to the blood vessels and heart, and it can increase your risk for a heart attack or stroke. That's why it is very important to treat the condition. Possible side effects of antihypertensive medicines are lightheadedness, dizziness, fatigue, drowsiness, confusion, insomnia, and nervousness. Each of these can impair driving performance, and people taking antihypertensives should be cautious about driving.

Some antihypertensive medications also have a diuretic effect, that is, they increase your need to urinate. This effect can interfere with safe driving, since you may need to use the bathroom more frequently. It can also lead to imbalances in your body chemistry, which can cause dizziness or fainting. People taking antihypertensive medication that has a diuretic effect should be especially cautious about driving.

Antipsychotics

Psychosis is a serious mental illness that involves distorted or unrealistic thinking, delusions, or hallucinations. Some common antipsychotic drugs are Risperdal® (risperidone), Zyprexa® (olanzapine), Haldol® (haloperidol), and Thorazine® (chlorpromazine). Almost all antipsychotic medications can significantly impair driving ability. These drugs can cause drowsiness, which is sometimes severe. They can also affect the central nervous system and interfere with a person's ability to think clearly or control movement. A person taking antipsychotic medications who experiences any of these symptoms should not drive.

Benzodiazepines (sedatives)

Benzodiazepines are primarily used to treat anxiety, but they are sometimes prescribed for other reasons such as to relax muscles, to treat seizures or panic disorders, and to induce sleep. Benzodiazepines are sedatives that slow down the central nervous system. They can impair driving because they affect vision, attention, and motor coordination. Some common benzodiazepines are Ativan® (lorazepam), Halcion® (triazolam), Klonopin® (clonazepam), Valium® (diazepam), and Xanax® (alprazolam). The effects of these medications can linger long after they're taken. For instance, even if they are taken at night, they can still impair a person's driving ability the next day. This is especially true for older people or anybody who uses alcohol. People taking sedatives should use extreme caution when considering whether or not to drive. If you take long-acting sedatives, or if you take sedatives during the day, you should not drive.

Muscle Relaxants

Muscle relaxants, such as Flexeril® (cyclobenzaprine) and Soma® (carisoprodol), are used to relax stiff, sore, or injured muscles. Muscle relaxants affect the central nervous system, and they can have a serious effect on driving safety. Muscle relaxants can cause drowsiness, dizziness, blurred vision, clouded thinking, weakness, and lack of coordination. People taking muscle relaxants should not drive when they first begin taking the medication. Even after a period of adjustment to the medication, those who take muscle relaxants should be very cautious about driving.

Narcotic Analgesics (opioids)

Narcotic analgesics, or opioids, are used to treat pain. One common opioid, codeine, is also often used to reduce coughing. If you are taking cough medicine, check the label to see if it contains codeine or hydrocodone, which is another opioid.

In the U.S., opioids are available only by prescription. These drugs affect the central nervous system and have a strong sedating effect. They can cause drowsiness, dizziness, and an exaggerated sense of well-being. It is very dangerous to drive while taking opioids. One of the most common opioids is morphine, which is the active ingredient in many brand-name prescription medications. Other common brand-name opioids are: Demerol® (meperidine), Dilaudid® (hydromorphone), OxyContin® (time-released oxycodone), Percocet® (oxycodone and acetaminophen), Tylenol #3® (acetaminophen and codeine), and Vicoden® (hydrocodone and acetaminophen). People taking these or any other opioids should not drive.

Nonsteroidal Anti-inflammatory Drugs

Nonsteroidal anti-inflammatory drugs, or NSAIDs, are used to treat swelling, joint and muscle pain, arthritis, and other related conditions. Some NSAIDs can be bought over the counter in the form of ibuprofen (Advil®, Motrin®) and naproxen (Aleve®). Other NSAIDs are only available by prescription.

Over-the-counter NSAIDs seem to pose little risk to driving when taken according to the label guidelines. However, recent research has indicated that certain prescription NSAIDs may increase the risk of heart attack and stroke, which in turn could endanger you when driving. This risk has so far been clearly associated only with certain prescription NSAIDs. If you are taking a prescription NSAID, you should talk to your doctor about its potential to impair your driving ability.

Parkinson's Disease Medications

Among the drugs sometimes prescribed to treat Parkinson's disease are Permax® (pergolide), Sinemet® (carbidopa and levodopa), and Symmetrel® (amantadine). Some of the common side effects of antiparkinsonian drugs are extreme sleepiness in the daytime, lightheadedness, blurred vision, and confusion. People taking antiparkinsonian drugs who experience any of these symptoms shouldn't drive. Parkinson's disease by itself can interfere with safe driving, since it can cause shakiness and stiffness, as well as a lack of muscle control, balance, and coordination. People with Parkinson's disease should be evaluated by a driver rehabilitation specialist to determine whether or not it's safe for them to drive.

Stimulants

Stimulants that are approved for medical use are prescribed to treat certain conditions such as attention deficit/hyperactivity disorder (ADHD) and sleep disorders such as narcolepsy. Some commonly prescribed stimulants are Adderall® (dextroamphetamine and amphetamine), Dexedrine® (dextroamphetamine), Provigil® (modafinil), and Ritalin® (methylphenidate). Some of the side effects of these drugs are headache, insomnia, anxiety, irritability, overconfidence, and general feeling of being "high." Each of these symptoms can interfere with driving safety. People should not drive during the initial stages of taking stimulants. Even after a period of adjustment to the medication, those who take stimulants should be very cautious about driving. Stimulants have a high potential for abuse, and people who abuse them or take more than the amount prescribed by a doctor shouldn't drive.

Vitamins and Minerals

The Harvard School of Public Health defines vitamins very simply: "Vitamins are nutrients you must get from food because your body can't make them from scratch." Minerals are what our teeth and bones are made of, and they are also something that our bodies can't make on their own. Experts agree that it's better to get vitamins and minerals from food rather than from supplements. However, some people need to take supplements due to a condition or illness. For instance, many older people need to take vitamin or mineral supplements in order to ensure proper nutrition.

Vitamins and minerals aren't dangerous unless you ingest too much of them, and it's nearly impossible to get too many just from the foods you eat. But if you take vitamin supplements, it's possible, even easy, to overdo it. Sometimes, taking too much of a vitamin or mineral can lead to problems ranging from an upset stomach to blurred vision to nerve damage. These side effects can impair driving performance. Taking too much of a vitamin or mineral can also interfere with how certain medications work, and this, too, can lead to problems with driving safely. Ask your healthcare provider if you should take any vitamins or minerals.

Herbal Supplements

Herbal supplements have become very popular in the last few years, and claims for their health benefits are common and sometimes outrageous, though largely unproven by rigorous scientific research. Some herbs can be beneficial, but others can be harmful. It is important to talk to your doctor before you start taking any herbal supplements. Herbal supplements can be like drugs in that they can affect our mental and physical conditions. They can cause serious medical problems if used incorrectly or if taken in large doses. They can also interact with other prescription or over-the-counter medications. For example, ginkgo, a herb taken in the hope of preserving cognitive function, interacts with aspirin. The interaction places a patient at risk for a brain bleed. Obviously, in such cases, taking herbal supplements can have a negative impact on driving safety.

Keep in mind that just because an herbal supplement is labeled "natural" doesn't mean it is safe. According to the National Institutes of Health (NIH), some herbs have been shown to be harmful. Kava and comfrey have been linked to serious liver damage. In addition, as the NIH Web site states, "In the United States, herbal and other dietary supplements are regulated by the U.S. Food and Drug Administration (FDA) as foods. This means that they don't have to meet the same standards as drugs and over-the-counter medications for proof of safety, effectiveness, and what the FDA calls Good Manufacturing Practices." As a result, sometimes what is inside the bottle is not the same thing as what is printed on the label. Thus, the need for open and honest communication with your healthcare provider and pharmacist is clear.

Tips for Taking Medications Safely

The Agency for Healthcare Research and Quality (AHRQ) has made patient medication safety a national priority. AHRQ recommends the following tips for taking your medicines safely.

BE INFORMED ABOUT YOUR MEDICATION.

Ask questions if you have doubts or concerns about your medicine. Questions to ask your healthcare provider or pharmacist before you take your medication include

1. What is the brand name and generic name of this medicine?

2. Can I take the generic version of this medicine?

3. What am I taking this medicine for?

4. Does this new prescription mean I should stop taking any other medicines I'm taking now?

5. How often do I take the medicine? If I need to take it three times a day, does that mean to take it at breakfast, lunch, and dinner or to take it every 8 hours?

6. Do I need to take it all or should I stop taking it when I feel better?

7. How long will I be taking it? Can I get a refill? How often can I get a refill?

8. Are there any tests I need to take while I'm on this medicine?

9. When should I expect the medicine to start working? How can I tell if it's working?

10. Are there foods, drinks (including alcoholic beverages), other medicines, or activities to avoid while I'm taking this medicine?

11. When should I tell the doctor about a problem or side effect?

12. What are the side effects that can occur with this medicine?

13. What should I do if I have a side effect?

14. What happens if I miss a dose?

15. What printed information can you give me about this medication?

GIVE YOUR HEALTHCARE TEAM IMPORTANT INFORMATION.
As mentioned earlier in the chapter, be sure to tell your healthcare providers about all the medicines, vitamins, herbal remedies, and dietary supplements you are taking every time you see them.

Stay with your treatment plan.

Nearly half of us don't follow our treatment plan as prescribed. The medicines may have side effects that are unpleasant or we may feel better and stop taking a medication early. This can be hazardous. For example, stopping an antibiotic too early can cause the more resistant strains of a bacteria to multiply, leading to a more serious and difficult-to-treat infection. It is important to stick with your treatment plan, and to tell your doctor if you are unable to do so.

Keep a record of your medications.

A record can help you keep track of your medications. Be sure to add new medicines to the list when you start something new or when you change your dose. Show the list to your doctor and pharmacist and make a copy for your family or a trusted friend in case of emergency.

CHAPTER 4

Planning to Avoid Dilemmas

Experts in the field of aging advise that we should invest the same level of preparation and thought in planning for our long-term mobility as we do in planning for our retirement. In other words, you should put as much time and energy into making plans for how you will get around when you get older as you do in preparing your finances, insurance, and living situation. That's advice few people have heard, and even fewer have heeded. But the guidelines offered in this chapter will allow you to act on this advice and start planning for your future mobility or that of a loved one.

Of course, it's likely that you are reading this book because you have to deal with a driving issue right now or will need to do so in the very near future. If you or a loved one hasn't made mobility plans, this chapter will be of great use to you. It will help you set the stage for talking with an older person about driving, assessing that person's driving fitness, and determining the best course of action for *everyone* involved. The chapter is addressed to people who are concerned about an older driver, but its contents will also be helpful to you if you are concerned about your *own* driving.

It's hard for many people to talk about this subject because it strikes at some powerful emotions surrounding independence, competency, and personal freedom. But delaying talking about the issue can be problematic or even dangerous, as illustrated in the tragic Santa Monica case study described in Chapter 1. This chapter will give you some critical information that will go a long way to reducing the discomfort of bringing up the subject and the uncertainty of how to handle possible scenarios.

Listed below are the general steps for developing a plan to deal with issues related to driving fitness. They are more fully described later in the chapter. You may find it helpful to keep a notepad and pen beside you for jotting down your thoughts as you consider the questions asked at many of the steps.

Planning Steps

    1. Get in the proper mindset.

    2. Start talking about driving safety.

    3. Screen for problems.

    4. Interpret the screening results and, if necessary, make further assessments.

    5. If necessary, get an assessment from a certified driving rehabilitation specialist.

    6. Make a plan for the driver to resume, remediate, rehabilitate, restrict, or stop driving.

    7. Keep talking and, if driving continues, keep monitoring the situation.

    8. Take care of yourself.

Step One: Get in the Proper Mindset

The first step is to get yourself in the proper mindset for a discussion about driving. Make sure that you know what your reasons are for bringing up the subject with an older driver. Also, even though your feelings and interests are important, the conversation shouldn't be about you. Your focus should be on the goals of keeping the driver as safe *and* independent as possible. Keeping these twin goals in mind will allow you to plan, speak, and act in a way that communicates your genuine concern and love.

In addition, understand that the idea is to work *together* to come up with a proper solution to the driving dilemma at hand: don't feel as if you're the one dictating what happens to someone else. Above all, keeping a caring, positive attitude is essential to fostering good interactions with the driver you are worried about. It will help you enlist the driver in problem solving with you, and it will help minimize negative emotional fallout.

- *Tip*: Don't approach this situation as though you're the only one making decisions or as though all the responsibility and burden rests on you. Instead, approach it as if you and the older driver are working *together* to solve a problem about his or her mobility needs and any driving safety risks.

- *Question*: What's your motivation in wanting to talk about and assess this person's driving abilities?

- *Question*: What scares you about this situation?

- *Question*: What is the worst thing that could happen if you *do not* address the driving dilemma?

- *Question*: What's the worst thing that could happen if you *do* address the driving dilemma?

- *Question*: What is the best thing that could happen if you address the issue?

- *Question*: What can you do to keep the proper mind-set and to stay focused on the goal of keeping the driver as safe *and* independent as possible?

Step Two: Start Talking About Driving Safety

Ideally, you'll have a long history of honest, frank communication with the older driver you are concerned about. In a perfect situation, you would have talked about health, housing, money, driving, and end-of-life care long before they become issues. However, in the real world, most of us delay or avoid addressing these problems until we absolutely have to.

Think about when and how you will first approach the topic of driving safety with the driver. I encourage you to read Chapters 6 and 7 which have in-depth information on communication techniques that can help you get started. Don't begin with a heavy or detailed conversation. The first time you talk about the subject should be just a brief, very general conversation about driving. What you want at this step is simply to establish driving as a legitimate topic of conversation. It *is* something many families talk about.

Below are a few examples of conversation starters for that first conversation. Realize that it will take *many* conversations about driving to resolve the dilemma and stay committed to having those conversations, no matter how long it takes.

- You could ask the older driver to tell you about learning to drive. Get the story of it all—for instance, how old was he or she;

what kind of car was it; who taught him or her, etc. I found these old stories to be wonderful pieces of family history that I had no idea about until asking.

• If your loved one is especially frugal or on a tight budget, check with AARP or AAA for reports about the high annual costs for maintaining an automobile. Then you could say something like, "*Wow, this AAA study found that in 2004 on average it cost $7,834 a year to own and operate a car.*"

• In a non-driving situation, bring up a news report of an accident involving an older driver, thus raising the subject without putting the person on the defensive. Sometimes it is clear from news reports that a particular driver was functionally impaired or that the vehicle mechanically failed in some way. These are specific issues that can be discussed in reference to the article. For instance, you might say, "*According to this article, more than 20% of people over age 65 have an uncorrected vision problem. That's a lot of people who can't see very well driving around.*"

You may find that the driver or some members of your family can easily anticipate where this discussion is eventually going and become visibly uncomfortable. Starting slowly and modestly will break the ice and introduce driving safety in the conversation. Talking about tough issues is a *process*. One conversation isn't going to be enough. At this point, all you are trying to do is to get the ball rolling. If family members resist or are openly hostile to these very general discussions, don't push it yet. Just make your general point, get the topic out there, and let the conversation go where it will. You'll learn in Chapters 6 and 7 how to handle some of the tougher conversations. At this stage, you are just getting the topic on the radar screen in a very general, nonjudgmental way. If the driver has a strong negative reaction to the initial, very general discussions, that will help you to know how to prepare for the later, more in-depth conversations.

• *Tip*: Think about when and how you will break the ice. You might want to bring up the topic in the car, but you should do so only if *you* are driving, not the person you are concerned about. Or you might want to talk about it after you have returned from a trip together, or after you have first arrived at the person's home.

• *Tip*: Be patient. Although some people will be open to talking about driving, others will resist. It may take some time and several tries to get a conversation going. Don't give up.

Step Three: Screen for Problems

Once you've broken the ice about driving, complete the Warning Signs screening form described in Chapter 1 and included in Appendix 1. Filling out this form will help you determine if your loved one has any of the common driving safety risks. This form will help you to provide feedback to the driver and can also help you engage the driver in a conversation about driving. If possible, ask the driver to complete the Driving Safety Quiz in Appendix 1. You can complete a Driving Safety Quiz about your own driving and compare results. Doing so may make a conversation about driving easier, since you can focus on something concrete together. Having objective results can make the whole process seem less personal and uncomfortable, both for you and for the driver.

In addition to filling out assessment forms, it is also important to ride in the car with the person and observe his or her actual driving performance. Research suggests that older drivers are more willing to listen to those who have actually driven with them. When you ride with the older driver, note specific instances of driving safety risks, but, if at all possible, don't point them out while the person is driving. Having a critical backseat driver can make even the most competent driver nervous or annoyed. Document your concerns after the drive is over. Your notes can provide useful, detailed information about what's wrong.

Remember, safe drivers need to **see, think,** and **move** well. Your observations and notes can help you determine which, if any, of these three functions is impaired. In addition, answers on the screening forms should point to whether the problems are related to seeing, thinking, or moving or to some combination of them. When you know what function is impaired, the course for further assessment and eventual intervention becomes clearer. Proper interventions may correct a problem enough for driving to continue on a limited basis.

- *Tip*: Photocopy the Warning Signs screening form and Driving Safety Quiz in Appendix 1.

- *Tip*: Review Chapter 1 to understand why the warning signs indicate a potential problem.

- *Tip*: Be considerate when evaluating the person's driving performance. Don't be judgmental, and remind the person that you are not judging but providing feedback and acting out of love and concern for him or her.

- *Tip*: Take your time with the evaluations, providing feedback and talking about the results with the older driver. You don't need to do this all in one day.

Step Four: Interpret the Results of Screening Forms and, If Necessary, Make Further Assessments

Next, review the screening form and self-assessment form. What, if any, problems were identified? Do the warning signs seem to have a pattern? Is it obvious that the problem is related to seeing, thinking, moving, or some combination? What is the level of risk (red, yellow, green)? Based on your answers to these questions, further assessment may be needed.

If the screening forms indicate a slight risk, consider getting the AAA Roadwise Review™ program described in Chapter 1 for more detailed assessment information. I think the positive approach of the program, its low cost, and the privacy of results make it an excellent tool for assessing driver skills at the next level.

If the screening forms indicate that the older driver has a problem with vision, schedule an appointment with an eye doctor as soon as possible. A visit to the eye doctor is usually not perceived as a big threat to independence, so it should be relatively easy to get the driver to make such a visit. If possible, drive the person to the eye doctor because the exam should include a dilated pupil exam that leaves eyes very sensitive to light and glare.

Quite a few vision problems can be corrected, allowing a person to continue to drive safely. However, others may require modifying driving habits (such as only driving during the daytime) or quitting driving altogether. A doctor's diagnosis of a vision problem can actually be helpful to the older person's attitude. Being able to cite a diagnosed vision problem can help the older person to retain some dignity if he or she has to limit or stop driving. Another reason to accompany your loved one on this visit is to get to know the eye doctor. If there is a serious vision problem, you may need to ask him or her to submit a letter or form to your state's Department of Motor Vehicles. A report from a physician is enough to trigger licensing actions (request for formal assessment, limitation, or suspension). This reporting process is described further in Chapter 5.

If it appears that the problem involves thinking or moving or some combination of causes, it is time to get a comprehensive medical evaluation as described in Chapter 1. It may be difficult at first to persuade an older person to see a doctor, but don't give up. If there is a Geriatric Assessment Clinic available in your area, try to schedule an appointment there. Most medical schools have these highly specialized clinics. To get an appointment, you may call directly or ask the primary care physician to make a referral. The advantage of a geriatric assessment is that it is a comprehensive, multi-disciplinary examination conducted by professionals who have undergone extensive training in diagnosing and treating older adults. So, for example, the driver's cognitive status may be evaluated by a geropsychologist or neurologist; physical function by a geriatrician or geriatric nurse practitioner; and available social resources by a geriatric social worker. You may communicate your concerns to the clinical team before the visit. Again, I suggest you try to accompany your loved one to the visit. These professionals can be a big help to you and your loved one.

- *Question*: What is the name and address of the driver's eye doctor? Do the screening results indicate a problem with vision? When was the last appointment? If more than 12 months ago, schedule a visit.

- *Question*: What is the name and address of the driver's primary care physician? Is this physician comfortable evaluating for driving fitness? Call to find out. Mention that you are concerned about driving fitness and want to schedule a medical evaluation.

• *Question*: Is there a Geriatric Assessment Clinic available in your area? Is the primary care physician familiar with it?

• *Tip*: Don't be reluctant to seek a comprehensive geriatric assessment. It takes the burden off you and the driver and puts it in objective, experienced hands.

• *Tip*: Emphasize the importance of maintaining good health in general, and, if necessary, downplay the connection between a doctor's visit and driving issues.

Step Five: If Necessary, Get an Assessment from a Certified Driving Rehabilitation Specialist

If assessments by screening forms, an eye doctor, primary care physician, or geriatrician have made clear what needs to be done about the older person's driving, then you can skip to Step Six. However, if these resources haven't resolved the driving safety risks, now is the time to contact a driving clinic and arrange to have your loved one assessed by a certified driving rehabilitation specialist. Appendix 3 has information on how to find and access such programs, and the communication style of motivational interviewing described in Chapters 6 and 7 should help you discuss this option.

The professional driving assessment will determine what problems exist and will offer solutions whenever problems can be corrected. The assessment will also provide resources and advice if problems *can't* be corrected.

• *Tip*: You or someone else should accompany the driver to the professional assessment. This can be a scary process, and having a loved one close by often helps.

Step Six: Make a Plan for the Driver to Resume, Remediate, Rehabilitate, Restrict, or Stop Driving

Work with the driver to make a plan to follow the recommendations given by the professional(s) who performed the formal assessment(s). The assessment professionals should provide you with written results of the exam and guidance for the future. Of course, the specific recommendations will vary according to each person's mental and physical conditions. It's possible that the driver can continue driving without restriction. On the other hand, maybe the person has to undergo driver retraining, or address some physical problem, such as getting a new prescription for eyeglasses, before returning to driving. Similarly, some kind of physical rehabilitation or modification to the car may be required in order to return to safe driving. Chapter 8 describes a few of the many common assistive devices that are available to help. For some people, the recommendation will be to restrict driving to certain times of day or to certain roads, while for others the recommendation will be to stop driving altogether.

If driving restrictions or retirement are indicated, determine what alternative transportation options will be needed to maintain quality of life. Make a list of options that the older person could and would realistically use. These might include public transit, taxicabs, services provided by private companies or volunteer organizations, or willing family or friends. It's important to make it clear that you're working together to help solve the problem of mobility.

Chapters 6 and 7 will help you to communicate empathically during this planning. In time, the driver may want to discuss what to do with the vehicle. It can be sold, given away, or donated to charity. Donating the car can provide some people with a profitable tax deduction. Some innovative programs, such as the Independent Transportation Network (which started in Maine and is now expanding nationwide as ITN America), accept donated cars and apply the value of the car to an older person's travel account, which can then be used to purchase rides. Another issue you'll need to address, if the person's driver's license has to be surrendered, is identification. Many Departments of Motor Vehicles offer photo identification cards free or at low cost, and you'll want to make an appointment to get one of those. If driving retirement is indicated due to cognitive impairment, determine if alternative housing and care options are needed.

- *Question*: What are the transportation options available if the person has to stop driving? Identify all the options, including public transportation, taxicabs, private services, services provided by religious or volunteer organizations, and the realistic capacities of willing friends and family.

- *Tip*: Contact the aging services professionals in your area. Appendix 3 has a listing of aging resources. These organizations are likely to have an informational and referral service that can help identify resources to keep your loved one as mobile as possible.

Step Seven: Keep Talking, and, If Driving Continues, Keep Monitoring the Situation

Even after a decision is made, it's important to keep the lines of communication open. People who stop driving need help working out their transportation needs, but just as importantly they may need emotional support. Contrary to what you might expect, people report feeling mostly sad, rather than angry, when forced to restrict or give up driving. Be sensitive to the emotions involved. Keep in mind that, while the decision to stop driving may be a onetime event, there are certain to be unexpected consequences or challenges down the line. Your help and understanding will allow former drivers to meet those challenges with dignity.

A person might agree to stop driving, but then renege on that agreement. Don't get overly alarmed because that's not unlike someone who has decided to break a bad habit, but then relapses. Read Chapter 6 to review how to handle resistance and acknowledge the difficulty of making any sort of major change.

However, if the person has become cognitively impaired and doesn't understand, you may have to take some extra, less direct measures, such as hiding the car keys or disabling the car. The older person may not have the capacity to decide to limit or stop driving and to follow through with it.

If the decision is that the older person can continue driving safely, you should keep monitoring the situation. Be especially attuned to any changes in the person's physical or mental condition that could affect driving. If the person's driving is now limited, find out if alternative transportation options are working out as needed. If assistive devices are required, determine whether the driver is using them correctly and comfortably.

- *Tip*: Enlist the support of your family and any healthcare providers involved. Having the help and ideas of many will help smooth the person's transition from the driver's to passenger's seat.

- *Tip*: Remember that driving fitness and performance can change over time. If new risks arise, you'll need to talk with the driver and reassess driving fitness.

Step Eight: Take Care of Yourself

Recognize that this can be an emotionally draining process. The stresses of caregiving are very real and can lead to physical or emotional problems of your own. Make taking care of your own health and fitness as much a priority as caring for a loved one. You can't help anyone else if you are incapacitated by stress. Talk often to supportive people. Get enough rest. Eat healthy foods and do everything you can to keep your health, fitness, and emotional condition at their peak.

- *Tip*: Plan each week so that you leave enough time to exercise regularly, get enough sleep, and eat well.

- *Tip*: Talk regularly with supportive friends or other family members about the situation. Ask others to help you communicate with and support the older person, including providing transportation, if they can.

- *Tip*: Find ways to do things that replenish your spirit. Make time to do things that bring you peace.

Resolving the driving dilemma is seldom simple or quick, but you *can* do it. This chapter described the overall process and gave you some tips to implement at the various stages in the journey.

In later chapters you'll learn communication strategies that will help you to be both caring *and* effective as you and your loved one deal with this issue. Keep the focus on safety and maintaining as much mobility and independence as possible. If you find yourself being drawn into negative emotions such as anger, frustration, or hurt feelings, stop, step back, cool down, and regroup. Proceeding from positive emotions will help everyone involved make the right decisions, work as a team, and reduce the chances of lingering resentments or other relationship problems.

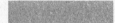

CHAPTER 5

Legal Issues and License Regulations

Driving is so universal in the U.S. that it's easy to view it as some kind of fundamental right—like freedom of speech or the right to a fair trial. In fact, driving is a *privilege* that is granted by a given state on the condition that the driver obeys various traffic laws and is capable of safely operating a vehicle. The state—and thus the law—can play an important role in any decision to limit or stop driving.

Currently there are no national laws about licensing older drivers. Each state makes its own regulations, which makes it a bit challenging to determine how your situation is affected by the law. I've tried to make it easier by including an updated state-by-state summary of regulations and medical standards for driving fitness, first assembled by the American Medical Association and the National Highway Traffic Safety Administration, in Appendix 3. In addition, Appendix 3 also has the name and address of each state's regulatory agency. The laws and regulations may have changed since this book was written, so be sure to check with your state regulatory agency—most have the information available on the

Internet. Ignorance of these laws can make an already complicated situation more difficult and contentious.

This chapter will explain the basis of driving-related laws and how to work with the appropriate regulatory agency (usually a state Department of Motor Vehicles). First, I will briefly review some of the key terms related to planning for later life (elder law), which can apply to issues of driving safety. If you have a family attorney, he or she may be able to assist you with your advance planning needs. This chapter will also describe typical procedures for reporting a potentially unsafe driver.

Elder Law: Planning Ahead

Elder law is fairly broad and covers fields such as:

- Disability planning, including use of durable powers of attorney, living trusts, living wills, and other means of delegating decision-making in case of incapacity.

- Social Security, Social Security Disability, and other retirement benefits.

- Wills and trusts that facilitate the transfer of property to beneficiaries.

- Medicaid and Medicare.

Like any branch of law, elder law is full of complexities that can most effectively be handled by an attorney who specializes in this field. If the cost of an attorney is beyond your means, however, you can probably find advice and help from public agencies such as local departments on aging, local senior centers, or some of the nonprofit organizations listed in Appendix 3. Another low-cost option might be found at your local law school. Check to see if a law school has a law clinic devoted to elder law staffed by advanced students who are supervised by a professor.

For any adult, it makes sense to identify a person who will be empowered to make decisions for you if you are ever incapacitated. You should do this whether or not you consult with an elder law attorney. (If you are concerned about an older person, you should talk with him or her about making such a decision.) Preparing for something you don't want to think about and certainly don't want to happen isn't comfortable or easy, but don't delay. It's important to make your wishes known so that they can be implemented should you become incapacitated.

Power of Attorney

A power of attorney is a document in which you give someone legal authority to act for you. This person is called your attorney-in-fact, and it should be someone you trust completely. You can control how broad the powers of your attorney-in-fact can be and can revoke a power of attorney at any time. A limited power of attorney gives the person authority to do only very specific tasks such as handling a particular financial matter. A power of attorney, however, becomes void if you become incapacitated, which is precisely when you would need someone to act on your behalf. This aspect of a power of attorney tends to make it an insufficient tool for planning for all of your future needs. The durable power of attorney is generally a better option.

Durable Power of Attorney

The durable power of attorney statute is a uniform law and is pretty much the same across states. There are two types of durable powers of attorney: one takes effect upon incapacity, and one is effective upon execution and is not revoked by incapacity. The great advantage of a durable power of attorney is that you are authorizing someone to act on your behalf even after you are incapacitated. However, designate only somebody you trust deeply because you are granting powers to control your money, your house, and (in the case of driving) your freedom to drive.

To plan ahead for a time when your driving fitness may be in question, you could note in your durable power of attorney document the circumstances by which you would surrender your license, cancel your car insurance, and dispose of your vehicle. In regard to determining driving fitness, you could stipulate that you want this process to include a professional assessment and express a willingness to abide by the findings of the professional evaluation. This is one proactive way to deal with the driving dilemma.

Healthcare Proxy

You should give someone the specific power to make healthcare decisions for you if you are unable to make these decisions. Many hospitals now require the designation of a healthcare proxy as a part of any admission. This includes the power to consent to the giving, withholding, or stopping of any medical treatment, service, or procedure. It is also possible to incorporate into this document the designation of someone you grant authority to make decisions about your driving.

Guardianship

In guardianship, the court appoints a person to perform certain court-ordered tasks. These tasks include caring for an incapacitated adult's financial affairs and personal needs. For handling only financial affairs, a conservatorship rather than guardianship is used.

Honestly, guardianship is the least desirable option for dealing with your potential incapacitation because of the expense and administrative burden involved. Unfortunately, it is the default option for people who haven't planned ahead. Having to appear in court before a judge to discuss sensitive personal information (such as your mental competence) is not high on the list of enjoyable activities for anyone.

Understanding State Regulations and Taking Action

Preparing in advance for driving restrictions or driving retirement is clearly the best option for everyone involved. Unfortunately, few people specifically address driving cessation in documents such as a durable power of attorney. If you are wrestling with a decision to limit or stop driving, try to learn about your state's laws related to this decision.

The need to familiarize yourself with the law becomes particularly acute if the driver suffers from moderate to severe cognitive impairments. If talking, reviewing screening forms, or getting advice from an eye doctor or other physician don't work, you may need to try more aggressive action—which means invoking the law. Drivers who pose a serious, documented risk to themselves or others require immediate attention, and you will need to work with the legal and regulatory systems to keep your loved one and the roads safe.

This section explains how to work with your department of motor vehicles. I describe the process to follow to report an unsafe driver (and include a sample letter to the DMV). State regulations can change, of course, so contact information for each state is included in Appendix 3 which will allow you to find out if the regulations have recently changed.

Working with Your Department of Motor Vehicles: The Massachusetts Example

Even though each state has its own specific rules about driving, most follow the same broad pattern of policies and procedures. I'm going to use my home state—Massachusetts—as an example in order to give you a sense of how most states work and provide a model for how to navigate the system in your state.

In most states, the agency that regulates driving is called the Department of Motor Vehicles (DMV). In Massachusetts, the state agency is called the Registry of Motor Vehicles (RMV), which is a part of the Executive Office of Transportation. Its regulations determine who can—and who cannot—legally operate a motor vehicle in the state.

Minimum Standards to Operate a Motor Vehicle

Throughout this book I've emphasized that the basic physical functions needed for safe driving are the ability to see, think, and move. Not surprisingly, the Massachusetts RMV Medical Affairs Board has established minimum standards for each of these functions, specifically addressing vision, loss of consciousness and seizure conditions, and cardiovascular and respiratory conditions. What follows are excerpts from the regulations (as of 2006) stipulating the minimum standards for driver licensing.

• SEE

"Visual acuity and horizontal peripheral field of vision standards . . . [of] at least 20/40 distant visual acuity . . . in either eye, with or without corrective lenses, and not less than 120 degrees combined horizontal peripheral field of vision . . . [People whose distant visual acuity is] between 20/50–20/70 . . . in *either* [italics by the author] eye, with or without corrective lenses, and not less than 120 degrees combined horizontal peripheral field of vision [are] eligible for a 'daylight only' license. . . . [All licensees] must be able to distinguish the colors red, green, and amber. . . . [Licensee must not] have unresolvable diplopia [double vision]."

- THINK

"Any licensee . . . who has experienced a seizure, [fainting,] or any other episode of altered consciousness which will or may affect the safe operation of a motor vehicle must voluntarily surrender his or her license, or be subject to suspension or revocation, until such time as that individual has remained episode free for at least six (6) months."

"Any licensee . . . who is medically determined to be a Class IV heart patient according to the American Heart Association (AHA) functional guidelines . . . is not eligible for a . . . license, [because they] may suffer symptoms of heart failure even at rest and therefore are unsafe to operate motor vehicles. . . . Any [individual] who has an implanted cardiac defibrillator (ICD) is not eligible [to drive] until six (6) months after such [a] device has been implanted. . . . If . . . the [device] has triggered, . . . the [licensee is] required to voluntarily surrender his or her license or be subject to suspension or revocation until . . . [six months of a] 'trigger-free' period [have passed]. . . . Any licensee . . . whose oxygen saturation level is 88% or less at rest or with minimal exertion, even with supplemental oxygen, is not eligible for a . . . license . . . [and must] voluntarily surrender his or her license. . . . [This poses] a significant threat of loss of consciousness, cognitive dysfunction, and risk of heart failure at any given time."

- MOVE

". . . [I]ndividuals who suffer from an arthritis condition so severe as to prevent them from performing self-care [the ability to perform activities of daily living, such as bathing, dressing, feeding oneself, toilet functions] may be functionally unable to operate a motor vehicle safely and therefore require an individual assessment of their operating ability in the form of a medical certification from a physician."

As these RMV regulations make clear, Massachusetts recognizes that driving fitness is a matter of physical and mental function, not age. These excerpts also show that Massachusetts, like most states, is very specific when it comes to establishing who can drive legally and who cannot. Knowing the laws in your state can help you resolve your own driving dilemma. For instance, if you have less than 20/40 vision or have seizures or any of the other impairing conditions described above, then the law makes it clear that you must stop driving. The ability to rely on concrete, objective standards such as state regulations can help you persuade a medically unfit driver to stop driving, and being able to cite such laws can help that person feel better about the decision.

Reporting Requirements and Making a Report

Making a report about the functional ability of a driver involves following certain steps. Though there are variations in these steps, the general pattern in most states is similar. Here again, I'll use Massachusetts as the example.

In Massachusetts, the first line of responsibility is with the licensee (that is, the driver). If a licensee has a medical condition he or she believes may affect the ability to operate a motor vehicle, that person *must* report such condition to the RMV and refrain from operating a motor vehicle until the condition is resolved. However, many residents of Massachusetts do not know when, why, or how this self-reporting should be done.

If an interested party, namely someone other than the licensee (a family member, physician, law enforcement official, neighbor, physical therapist, elder law attorney, etc.), wants to submit a report to the RMV about a potentially unfit driver, the report

- must be in writing and signed by the person making the report. It must include the name, address, and telephone number of the person making the report. Anonymous reports are not accepted.

- must identify the full name of the unfit driver and include at least one of the following: social security number, license number, date of birth, or address.

- must contain the reason for the complaint and/or a description of the purported functional limitation. (The screening forms in Appendix 1 could be attached to your letter.)

The RMV has a medical evaluation form that is available to physicians to use in reporting. Alternatively, the physician can submit a report to the RMV on his or her official letterhead. In that case, the report must also include the physician's signed name, address, telephone number, and Massachusetts Board of Registration in Medicine number.

Sample Reporting Letter

Here is an example of a letter expressing concern about a driver that could be submitted to a state department or registry of motor vehicles.

Date

Dear Director of Medical Affairs:

I am writing this letter to report a driver who I think is unsafe to operate an automobile. The driver is my great-aunt, Jane Smith, of 100 Commonwealth Avenue, Boston, MA 02118. Her date of birth is February 7, 1919. Jane Smith has severe arthritis, such that she has very limited mobility, a heart condition, and cataracts. In addition, in the past year she has become very forgetful. Her car has scrapes and dents that she hasn't noticed and can't explain. She has a slow reaction time and when I last rode with her it seemed as if she couldn't see pedestrians in the crosswalk until it was almost too late. I have attached a warning signs form to document the extent of her problems.

I've asked her to get a professional assessment at the driving clinic at Beth Israel Deaconess Medical Center, but she refused and is now angry with me. I am very worried that she may be injured in an accident or may hurt someone else because of her functional limitations.

My name is
Elizabeth Dugan
200 Commonwealth Avenue
Boston, MA 02118
My daytime telephone number is (555) 123-4567.

Please contact me if I can provide any additional information. Thank you.

Sincerely,

Elizabeth Dugan

RMV Response

I interviewed Mr. Todd Brown, J.D., the Director of Medical Affairs for the Massachusetts RMV, to learn how the state will respond to a report, such as the one above. Mr. Brown explained that when the state receives a report from a private citizen about a licensed driver who may be unfit due to an alleged physical or mental condition, the RMV will conduct an assessment of the driver's qualifications to operate a vehicle safely. The RMV usually sends a medical response letter to the driver that requests a medical evaluation from his or her physician about the person's reported condition and medical qualification to operate a motor vehicle safely. The form usually must be returned within 30 days. After evaluating the physician's report, the RMV may take one of several appropriate licensing actions, including supporting, suspending, or revoking the license. Before taking licensing action however, the RMV may further assess the individual's ability to drive safely by requiring a road test and/or assessment for adaptive equipment and license restrictions. While the RMV is evaluating driver fitness, a hold is placed on the license record so that a new license will not be reissued until the evaluation is completed. Unfortunately, this process is not always a smooth or fast one.

The process moves a bit faster when the report is from a physician or law enforcement official because in that case the RMV may initiate a licensing action directly, without seeking a physician's evaluation. (Thus, proof of the value of communicating with the healthcare professionals involved in your loved one's assessment and care.)

Here is a description of the licensing actions that the Massachusetts RMV may take:

1. No further action if it concludes there is no basis to the complaint.

2. Request that the individual take a competency road exam and/or an assessment for adaptive equipment and appropriate license restrictions.

3. Request that the individual voluntarily surrender his or her license. A person who voluntarily surrenders his or her license is eligible to receive a Massachusetts state identification card, free of charge. In addition, when a license is voluntarily surrendered, there are no negative insurance ramifications, and if the person's condition improves, and he or she can document his or her qualification to drive safely, the license may be restored to its former active status.

4. If the individual does not comply with the RMV's request to voluntarily surrender the license, the Medical Affairs office may notify the Driver Control Unit to schedule a hearing on the matter. If the Driver Control Unit does not find in favor the individual, the license may be revoked.

This is a reasonable process in theory. However, in actual practice a few problems exist. Mr. Brown acknowledged that the system is not as responsive as he would like—on the day we talked, the RMV had approximately 1,800 forms related to medical reporting to be processed by only two staff members. Imagine what the backlog will be as the population continues to age! Mr. Brown also noted that the RMV has encountered some physicians who are reluctant to provide an evaluation of driving fitness. This is understandable given the uncertainty about how to do it—the AMA clinical guidelines for this process were only published in 2003 and still are not widely disseminated or followed. In addition, physicians may have concerns about violating new federal privacy regulations and/or have worries about possible liability issues. Finally, many physicians do not want to risk alienating a long-term patient, especially one in need of careful monitoring of chronic conditions. These valid concerns show that our social structures (such as the medical system and the regulatory agencies) have yet to catch up with the reality of a rapidly aging society.

What to Do While Waiting for a Response from the RMV

As noted above, if a report is made by a physician or law enforcement official, the process tends to move more quickly than if it is made by a private citizen. However, it still can take some time to resolve. Use the communication techniques described in Chapters 6 and 7 to help deal with potential negative reactions of a reported driver.

For loved ones with cognitive impairment, there are limits as to how effective communication will be. Learning and practicing all of the communication techniques described in the next chapters will not be enough to make this a smooth process. In such cases where you can't collaboratively problem-solve but must act immediately to keep your loved one and public safe, you may have to take extralegal steps. *I want to stress that taking such steps is only warranted in limited cases with a driver who is clearly dangerous and medically unfit to safely operate a vehicle, but who does not understand that he or she must stop driving.* Families are limited only by their creativity. Some of the extralegal steps people have taken include disabling the car, hiding keys, getting the car towed for repairs (that are never completed), loaning the car to someone who never returns it, and so on. Again, taking these actions is only justifiable in the case of dealing with a driver who is obviously dangerous and who is cognitively impaired. Don't do this because you are squeamish about having frank conversations.

❖   ❖   ❖

Driving is a privilege that many of us will outlive by about a decade. That's why it's important to plan ahead for your mobility needs and know how to work with the regulatory agency in your state. In some cases, emergency steps are needed. Most of us will be able to discuss the problem and solutions. The next chapters will help you to communicate about driving restrictions or cessation in a positive, collaborative way.

CHAPTER 6

Learning to Talk About Change

The preferred approach is to talk early, often, and within the context of maintaining health and vitality for as long as possible. Older drivers should talk with their healthcare providers, spouses, and family members about their concerns and/or desires in the event they no longer can drive safely. And family members should have started talking early, before driving is a safety concern. Unfortunately, for most of us, communication occurs late and under pressure—when someone's driving safety is already in question. Many people tell me that dealing with this issue was extraordinarily stressful, uncertain, and sad. *Not one* has reported feeling adequately prepared.

This chapter will help you prepare to talk about the issue of driving in a way that will minimize the risk of emotional land mines. I describe *motivational interviewing techniques,* a counseling approach widely used to communicate about extremely difficult topics. These techniques can help you to discuss driving-related issues with a friend, spouse, parent, or other relative.

Express Empathy

Before you talk to your loved one, spend some time reflecting on what driving restrictions or cessation may mean to him or her. Understand *all* that driving represents and what a change in driving status may mean to his or her identity. Later life is filled with wonderfully rewarding benefits and, at times, painful indignities. There's apt to be a lifetime of memories associated with driving, including going on dates; driving to the hospital to have a baby; going to a child's sporting or musical performances; teaching *you* how to drive; going to work; driving to visit family at holidays and other special occasions; or driving to attend important work or social functions. Taken together, these memories may represent a lifetime of independence.

Put yourself in the position of the older driver and recognize that stopping driving can be a significant blow to one's ego and self-esteem. Anticipate the problems or difficulties that being without a car might involve. Can your loved one continue with treasured activities? Make it a point to investigate this beforehand. A colleague of mine took this notion to heart when he realized he had to talk about driving cessation with his father. For two weeks, he forced himself to get around without driving. He did this to heighten his sensitivity to what he was going to ask his father to endure—the hassle, frustration, and humiliation of having to rely on others to get to appointments, run errands, see friends, and pursue other leisure activities. It also forced him to explore all the local transportation options so that when he sat down to talk with his father, he could share his own experiences and candidly discuss the emotional and logistical aspects of becoming dependent on others for transportation.

Anticipate Emotions

Thinking and talking about limiting driving or driving cessation may cause resentment, fear, anger, or feelings of vulnerability. However, *sadness* is the most common emotion reported by drivers who have hung up the keys for good. This makes a lot of sense because it is a loss of independence and identity. Crying during or after a discussion isn't uncommon. Don't be overly alarmed by intense expressions of sadness since crying is a natural expression of emotion. But do pay attention if the sadness lingers for weeks and months; research suggests that driving cessation can be associated with depressive symptoms. Depression is not a normal part of aging—be alert to signs of depression. The symptoms include feeling guilty or worthless, nervous or empty, very tired and slowed down; not enjoying things the way you used to, feeling like life is not worth living, sleeping or eating more or less than usual, and having persistent headaches, stomach aches, or chronic pain. Seek medical assistance if these symptoms persist for 4 or more weeks.

Anxiety and *worry* are the next most common emotions. One woman facing driving retirement worried aloud:

> . . . *but how will I get around? My son lives across town and I only see him on Sundays . . . I don't want to be a burden. How will I get to the grocery store, the bank, the post office, and to my synagogue if I can't drive?*

Communicating empathy, identifying alternative transportation options, and working creatively together on a plan can help relieve this well-placed worry about the future. Plan to acknowledge the validity of anxiety and worry.

Anger is another emotion that might be expressed. An older driver may be angry at what's perceived to be your snooping in his or her business; angry at the change in family roles; angry about his or her physical condition and decline. The motivational interviewing technique, called rolling with resistance, discussed later in this chapter, can be helpful in dealing with anger.

Fear is another emotion that is frequently experienced, yet is less often articulated. The driver who must stop or limit his or her driving may be afraid of what this change means. "Will I become a burden? Am I losing control? Will I suffer a long, debilitating decline? Am I approaching death? Will I have to move into a nursing home?" Many of these thoughts may race through someone's mind, yet will remain unspoken. While you might see the conversation as being just about driving restrictions or cessation, the older driver may see it as involving many other issues. Be aware that the whole process may be a scary and complicated one for the older driver.

General Communication Tips

It's just common sense to bring up sensitive conversations at a time and place when you won't be interrupted and won't have to rush. Sitting comfortably where everyone is at the same eye level also helps. Being close enough to comfort with a soothing pat on the shoulder or reassuring touch is a good idea, as is having tissues handy in case tears are shed. Don't fall into the trap of rehashing old arguments or making the conversations about anything other than your love and concern for the driver's safety and the facts relating to their driving fitness.

Know the Alternatives

We all have essential transportation needs. Getting food, supplies, and medicines and going to medical appointments are the bare minimum. Of course, most of us want and deserve more than this minimum, and being able to socialize with family and friends and to participate in enjoyable activities contributes to the richness of our life. Plan to spend some time identifying the resources available in your community to meet the older person's mobility needs. You're not likely to use every one, but you'll want to know what all the options are so that your loved one has some choice about how to get around. Bear in mind that one option probably isn't going to fully meet all the transportation needs. Rather, it's likely that you'll have to patch together several options, which I discuss below. Try to find out how senior-friendly each transportation option is, especially if your loved one has some cognitive or memory problems. While most services are door-to-door, or curb-to-curb, many seniors need more help than that. In that case, the service model that's really needed is called an "arm-in-arm" approach, in which the transporter goes to the door and assists the rider to and into the vehicle, and then at the destination assists him or her out of the vehicle and into the destination. Unfortunately, there aren't many such services in operation yet.

Keep in mind that most of us are creatures of habit. Having to adapt to new modes of transportation may be met with resistance. Be patient, and do what you can to help ease the transition and to establish a regular schedule for the person who has had to limit or give up driving.

Family. The most common providers of rides are family members because this is usually most convenient, safe, and familiar. Are any family members nearby and willing to help? To what extent are they willing to help? Reciprocity, the natural give-and-take in relationships, is an important aspect of social relations. Is it possible for the older adult to do or give something in return for the rides? For example, one way to foster reciprocity is to allow the older person to treat for lunch or to pay for gas as they are able and willing. This helps the older retired driver to feel less like a burden on others and also can help family members to feel less put upon. If possible, the responsibility for transporting the older person should not fall to one family member. Share the responsibility with others. Draw up a regular weekly schedule, and be sure to plan for urgent situations. Also, don't look at this only in the short term; depending upon the older person's physical and mental health, family members could spend *years* providing rides.

Friends and neighbors. Another comfortable transportation option for many people is to get rides from friends or neighbors. Many families do not live in close proximity to each other, but relationships with neighbors and friends may be quite close and supportive. Are there friends or neighbors who might be available and willing to provide transportation? This was an option that worked out well for one older woman with a severe vision impairment who could no longer drive. She had lived in the same house for more than 40 years and loved her neighbors. There was a "young" retired neighbor who cut her grass in the summer, snow plowed her driveway in the winter, and was very willing to drive her around once a week for a small fee. This took the pressure off her son who lived across town and was busy juggling his own career and family responsibilities.

Local programs. Many types of transportation programs are run by local organizations such as senior centers, city or county departments on aging, religious organizations, and nonprofit groups. To find such resources, contact your local Area Agency on Aging (see Appendix 3) which may have a current list of the local transportation options. Determine what, if any, costs are associated and when (days of the week, time of day) rides are available. If the older driver is a member of a faith community, check to see if it offers transportation services to seniors and disabled members.

Paratransit. Specialized transportation services for disabled people who can't use regular public transportation services such as buses, streetcars, or subways are called paratransit systems. Such systems are provided by public transportation authorities as part of the requirements of the Americans with Disabilities Act. The most common program is a dial-a-ride program that provides door-to-door service. To use this service you usually must complete an application and provide documentation of the disability (from a physician or other qualified professional). Rides are scheduled in advance and depending on the service, may or may not be shared with another person. Although paratransit might work out well for some, this may not be a desirable option for other seniors. It may be that you think the transportation option is viable but your loved one does not. You'll have to respect the person's feelings and work together to find another solution.

Mass Transit. Public transportation services such as buses, streetcars, trains, or subways may be another option, although these services are not ones used by many seniors. Be realistic in evaluating if it's possible for your loved one to navigate the system, given the functional issues that are forcing retirement from driving. For example, if cognitively impaired, it's unlikely he or she can remember when the bus will come, where it will take the person, how much the fare is, or to physically navigate getting on and off the bus. If the older person is willing and able to take public transportation, you might offer to take a few rides with him or her at first to create familiarity with the routes, schedules, fares, and other practical matters.

Taxi. Taxicabs are an often-overlooked option. The advantage of calling a cab is that it is time-flexible, not usually a shared ride, and provides door-to-door service. At first glance, it may seem that using taxi services is too expensive. However, compared to the cost of buying and maintaining a car, and paying for gas and insurance, cabs are usually a great deal. Try doing a rough estimate of how much an older adult currently spends on the upkeep of a car and then calculate how many average-length cab rides that would pay for. Also find out if the cab service in your town offers assistance for older riders.

Private programs. Retail shopping centers, assisted living communities, adult day care facilities, or other private programs may offer transportation services. Find out what's available in your community and who is eligible to use the services. How expensive are rides? What is the area served?

Plan to Persist

Talking is a *process*. When you're planning to talk about a driving issue, bear in mind that one conversation seldom does the trick. Moving from unlimited driving to driving retirement can be a lengthy process and usually involves numerous conversations. You can't anticipate everything that will come up in a discussion, and options agreed upon in one conversation may need to be revisited in later conversations.

Dealing with Dementia and Cognitive Impairment

If you are dealing with a driver who has been diagnosed with dementia or other cognitive impairment, you face some additional challenges. The first is the *inevitability* of driving cessation. While the plan for the other, nondemented, older drivers may involve a series of steps—from driving shorter distances, to driving only familiar roads, to being a co-pilot, to letting others do more and more of the driving—the plan for demented drivers is 100% fixed: driving retirement. Remediation or assistive devices are not going to be effective solutions in these situations.

The second challenge is the *complexity* of dealing with someone who has a progressive brain disease. In time, dementia affects judgment, personality, memory, reaction time, problem solving, insight, and even sensory perception. Dementia will affect the person's ability to understand that there is a problem with driving, and this will make the conversations difficult.

Third, because the rate of impairment and the precise abilities impaired may differ for each individual, there isn't one right way to approach this. You'll have to decide what makes sense for your situation. Talking about transitioning out of the driver's seat may work with people who are only mildly impaired; in fact, they may welcome a chance to discuss this with you. Sometimes early in the disease people recognize they are "slipping" and are terribly frightened by it. Being able to talk openly about driving and about this decline may help them to feel less alone and fearful, and may foster useful discussions of other concerns as well. However, for adults with a moderate or severe impairment, especially those hell-bent on driving, more extreme steps may have to be taken to keep the person and the public safe. Recent preliminary research suggests that a driving cessation support group for individuals with dementia and their caregivers can be helpful in easing the transition.

Motivational Interviewing

Motivational interviewing will be most useful if you are working with an older driver who is cognitively intact. Motivational interviewing is a counseling technique developed in the early 1990s by two psychologists, Drs. William Miller and Stephen Rollnick. Their early work with this counseling style focused on adults with substance abuse and related problems. However, motivational interviewing has been used in a wide range of situations—such as helping patients to adhere to treatment regimens for diabetes, to lose weight, or to quit smoking. Motivational interviewing has been used successfully to help many people to change behavior. I saw this approach work firsthand in one large research study that I was involved with, called the Women's Health Initiative (WHI), in which motivational interviewing helped the study participants (older women) make significant long-term dietary changes.

Motivational interviewing is a brief, *nonconfrontational* way of helping someone to achieve a change in behavior. If you have tried to lose weight, exercise more, or quit smoking, you know how hard it is to change any behavior—it takes motivation, effort, and support. For a driver who is no longer safe to drive, driving restriction or driving retirement could and should be viewed as a type of behavior change. Accordingly, instead of thinking that you have to coerce or persuade the older driver to stop, think of yourself as trying to help *facilitate the change in behavior* (the person's transition from the driver's seat to the passenger's seat). It is an assumption of motivational interviewing that **the ultimate responsibility for the change rests with the older adult**. Having this perspective is going to change your entire approach to communication.

A key advantage of this approach is that it recognizes that we all have motivation and resistance to behavior change and that there are both positive and negative motivations to changing any behavior. When we *must* make a change, we tend not to think about all the sides of an issue. Instead, we do what we should do or must do. But when the choice to make the change rests with us, identifying the pros and cons of changing and not changing is a useful exercise. Taking this step can help us to hang on to our plan during times of stress or temptation (such as sneaking out to drive the car after agreeing to stop driving).

The chart below is one way to map out the reasons for and against the decision to stop driving. This is a way to work out the *decisional balance*, helping the driver to weigh the pros and cons of the change. The driver reflects on the change (in this example, it is someone who had to retire from driving due to vision impairment from macular degeneration). You can see that she felt both positive and negative motivations in changing her driving behavior.

Weighing the Pros and Cons

Julie is an 83-year-old widow who lives alone in a retirement community in Central Florida. She is a retired medical secretary and has two sons who are both retired and living in Connecticut. Her younger sister and brother-in-law live in the same retirement community and they see or talk to each other every day. Julie is a cancer survivor and has been having vision issues for the past several years. She was recently diagnosed with macular degeneration in both eyes of such severity that she had to surrender her license to drive.

Here is how she sketched out the pros and cons of stopping driving.

	Benefits/Pros	Costs/Cons
Making a change (stop driving)	Comply with the law	Loss of independence
	Not cause an accident	Not able to have control of my schedule
	Could give the car to grandson	Have to impose on others for rides
	Save on expenses	Have to admit to myself I have limits

	Benefits/Pros	Costs/Cons
Not changing (keep driving)	Have control of when I go out	My family would be appalled
	Wouldn't think of myself as dependent	Risk of causing an accident
		Get a ticket or arrested if caught
	Maintain status quo	Could get sued if I caused an accident

Julie found it freeing to acknowledge that she had ambivalent feelings about making this difficult change. Articulating the mixed feelings made it easier for her to decide to comply with the state's request for her to surrender her license. The costs of not changing outweighed what the benefit of not changing might be.

Feel free to photocopy the chart below, and ask the driver to think about the pros and cons of the decision to drive or not drive and to write them in the boxes. Getting them out in the open can help you to communicate about them.

	Benefits/Pros	Costs/Cons
Making a change		

	Benefits/Pros	Costs/Cons
Not changing		

Readiness to Change

You are likely, in fact almost certain, to observe signs of resistance in your conversations about driving cessation or restriction (such as interrupting, ignoring, arguing, and denying). Instead of being blindsided or frustrated by these reactions, engaging in motivational interviewing teaches you to *expect* resistance. There are pros and cons to the decision, and you should be prepared to acknowledge them and to help the person making the change to weigh them. Viewing change as a process that involves the five stages described on page 98 should help you to understand how to match your responses to the stage the person is in.

In research studies, we often ask people to indicate how *ready* they are to make the required behavior change (such as increasing physical activity). We do this because someone who hasn't even thought about making a change needs to hear a far different message than a person who has made the change and is now trying to maintain it. The following table illustrates the continuum of *readiness to change*, a theory of change developed by psychologists Drs. Carlo DiClemente and James Prochaska. This is one of the most widely used approaches to understanding behavior change, with decades of research supporting its effectiveness.

The box on the far left represents the *precontemplation* stage. A person in this stage hasn't even thought about making a change, isn't intending to take action in the near future, and may be uninformed or underinformed about the consequences of his or her behavior. In the *contemplation* stage, the person is considering making a change in the near future (usually 6 months). At this stage, the person is highly aware of the pros and cons and may feel ambivalent about the change. In the *preparation* stage the person is preparing to make the change and has a plan of action to change. Someone who is going to stop driving would, at this stage, be finding out about alternative transportation options and deciding what to do with the car. Next comes the *action* stage, in which the person is actually making the change. A person in this stage has made specific, deliberate changes in lifestyle within the past 6 months. Finally, in the *maintenance* stage of change, the person has made the change and is working to maintain it, working to prevent relapse, and is increasingly confident about the ability to continue the change.

One benefit of thinking about change in this way is that you can tailor your responses to the person depending on where he or she is in the change process. For example, someone who is contemplating making changes would benefit from motivational messages such as "You've always made good decisions about your health in the past and I know you'll do the same thing when it comes to deciding what to do about driving." On the other hand, the person who has made the change may not need motivation so much as support in sticking with the change such as help arranging rides to the grocery store or hair salon.

In your early conversations it may be helpful to ask your loved one to think about where they see themselves falling along the following continuum. If the person you're talking to is not comfortable with paper and pencil exercises, you can determine where his or her attitude falls just as well by asking. Pick what works best for your relationship and situation.

Haven't thought about changing. Not ready to change.	Thought about changing. Still unsure about whether to change.	Decided to change. Taking steps to get ready to change.	Actively trying to change.	Made change, trying to live with it.
(Precontemplation)	**(Contemplation)**	**(Preparation)**	**(Action)**	**(Maintenance)**

As a result of your ongoing conversations, the interventions of medical professionals, driving specialists, and perhaps regulators, this readiness to change can be expected to move through the five stages of change (shifting from left to right). For example, if your loved one is in the *precontemplation* stage, then you'll want to increase awareness of the issue. Feedback from the warning signs form and the self-assessment quiz and articles from AARP, AAA, or some other sources may be helpful. You want your loved one to start thinking about it. If the person is in the *contemplation* stage, he or she may be weighing the pros and cons, and you'll want to use the communication skills described below to help resolve the ambiguity of the decision. Those in the *preparation* and *action* stages will need emotional and logistical support in making the change.

Once you and your loved one have determined his or her stage of readiness to change driving behavior, you can talk some more about the person's feelings and attitude. Use motivational interviewing techniques described below to engage the older driver in a non-threatening, nonjudgmental, productive conversation.

The Motivational Interviewing Approach

While I don't expect you to master this counseling style just by reading this book, you *can* benefit from understanding the spirit of this approach and learning some of the techniques associated with it. If you'd like to learn more or to obtain formal training, check the Web site http://www.motivationalinterviewing.org for information. Here, I'll start by explaining the guiding principles and key techniques of the motivational interviewing approach.

Expressing Empathy

Empathy, in the counseling sense, is more than just feeling someone's pain. By expressing empathy, you're telling the person that you understand where he or she is coming from, and that you accept and understand that person. Empathic communication is nonjudgmental. You don't evaluate the rightness or wrongness of what the person is expressing, you just try to understand it. The principle is that when someone feels understood, the person is more open to change. Motivational interviewing counselors believe that in the process of being understood, one's feelings and ideas will change in a problem-solving, insight-producing, and conflict-reducing way. The person gets the message from you that he or she makes sense and is worthy of being taken seriously. This may take some work on your part, because chances are you feel you know *exactly* what the person ought to decide or do. But your job here is to step back and listen to how that person views the issue. Understand, drop your agenda, and just listen.

Support Self-efficacy

Self-efficacy is the belief that you can change and that change is possible. Remember that children's story about the little train going up the mountain ("I think I can, I think I can")? That's an example of self-efficacy. You want to help the person who is making the change develop a firm conviction that change *is* possible and that he or she can do it. Having confidence that you can make the change is half the battle in successful behavior change. Pointing out past successes can help someone to grow in confidence that a future change can be made. When it comes to giving up driving, it is important to believe that relying on others for transportation is viable and that it can become a new part of his or her lifestyle.

Roll with Resistance

Underlying the motivational interviewing approach is the principle of rolling with resistance. I think it is this principle that makes this approach particularly well suited to help you discuss driving. Instead of trying to argue point and counterpoint, which nearly always leads to frustration, motivational interviewing teaches you to *roll with the resistance*. It's not your responsibility to convince the person that resistance is "wrong" or "pig-headed." As you now know there are positive and negative motivations to change. Hearing about the negatives isn't threatening or awful. Arguing is counterproductive to the change process, and forcing the older driver to defend his or her position may actually cause more resistance and defensiveness. Instead of challenging statements point by point, your task is to listen, express empathy and use the speaker's "momentum" to further explore his or her view. There's ambiguity around the decision, so let the person express both sides of it. Sometimes getting it all out verbally or in writing helps clarify what is swirling around in one's mind.

Contrary to what you might expect, this approach tends to *decrease* resistance rather than increase it. Once people hear themselves express resistance, they may be better able to objectify it and see the flaws in the position, or at least see some alternative ways of viewing the situation. Remember that a behavior change, like driving cessation, is a *choice*. Even when ordered by the state to stop driving, the person has to *choose to comply*. It may not feel like much of a choice, but it is. The person may feel frightened by the idea of change, and expressing fear through resistance is normal. The beauty of the motivational interviewing approach is that it encourages the person making the behavior change to figure out his or her own solutions to the problem that have been expressed as resistance. In this approach, you and the driver are on the same side. Your job is to *listen* empathically and reflectively and to help the person weigh the pros and cons of *the decision*.

Develop Discrepancy

Developing discrepancy is a way of helping the person to see a discrepancy between where the driver is and wants to (or has to) be. For instance, the older driver may hold a strong personal moral value of being a good example to his or her children or grandchildren. One way of developing discrepancy would be to ask the person to consider how violating the law or a doctor's orders regarding driving matches up with the goal of being a positive role model.

Reflective Listening

Reflective listening entails giving feedback to another person by reflecting back to the speaker in a nonjudgmental way what you heard said. You don't simply repeat what the person said, but rephrase it to show the speaker that you are listening carefully and understand. It also shows the person that his or her ideas make sense, because you are able to state the same ideas in different words but still in a logical way. It can be very reassuring to know that our ideas and attitudes are reasonable. By the same token, it can be very enlightening to hear someone else restate our thoughts in new words. We might understand those thoughts differently or realize they are not true reflections of what we want.

I had to attend a workshop on reflective listening a few years ago for work and, at first, cynically thought it sounded like a very phony technique. I couldn't fathom how parroting back words to someone would ever be helpful in any way. Toward the end of this workshop we paired off to practice what we had been learning. We each had to pick one behavior we wanted to change. The other person was to practice listening reflectively, summarizing, and rolling with resistance. I was out of shape and overweight and wanted to start exercising regularly again. So I had to express what my desired behavior change was (to exercise regularly), and what the pros (feel better; be healthier; lose weight) and cons (I was busy at work; I had moved and didn't have my workout partners anymore; I didn't belong to a gym, etc.) about making the change were. After the practice session, I found myself *really* getting motivated to make a change. When I heard my negative motivations reflected back to me nonjudgmentally and in slightly different words, they sounded so lame! I felt that the person practicing with me perfectly understood what I said and wasn't judging me; she just wanted to understand what the issues were. The process helped me to get unstuck and move forward in my readiness to change. Despite my initial skepticism, I found that when reflective listening is done right, it doesn't feel or sound phony at all; instead, it is a very affirming and clarifying communication tool.

Here's an example of a *simple reflection* related to driving:

Older driver: But I can't quit driving. I've got to get around!
You: Quitting driving seems impossible because you wouldn't be able to get where you want to go.
Older driver: Right. But maybe I should quit because my doctor told me it's not safe for me to drive anymore.

Here you have restated the older driver's concerns, allowing the person to take the next step and express a new idea. Instead of you reminding the older driver about the doctor's advice, the older driver has done so himself.

In *double-sided reflection*, you reflect the contradictory comments that express both the positive and negative side of the be-havior change:

> **Older driver:** My doctor told me it's not safe for me to drive anymore. But I can't quit driving. I've got to get around!
>
> **You:** You can't imagine how you will get where you want to go, and at the same time you respect your doctor and don't want to drive if you are not able to.
>
> **Older driver:** Yes, I've really got mixed feelings about this.

Here you help the older driver to see that the issue is complicated and that a simple solution or narrow view is not appropriate to dealing with it. It also validates the driver's feelings of ambivalence and can help the older person to grant as much value to reasons for quitting as to reasons for not stopping or limiting driving.

An *amplified reflection* is one I think best left to professionals because it's easy to sound sarcastic doing this. But I'll include an example so you can see the full range of reflections. In amplified reaction, you exaggerate what someone has said to the point where the person would disagree. This reflection can easily come across as patronizing, so be careful if you decide to use one.

> **Older driver:** But I can't quit driving. I've got to get around!
>
> **You:** So you are a safe driver who wants to go wherever and whenever you want to.
>
> **Older driver:** No, I just want to be able to take care of my own needs.

The idea of amplified reflection is to get the other person to be more concrete about his or her ideas. Again, though, it is not an approach I recommend you take, given the risks of sounding as if you're mocking or belittling the person.

Reframing is another related technique. In reframing, you ask the person to examine their perceptions in a new way. For example, suppose the older driver reports that a relative said, "You really need to see a doctor about your driving" and the person views this as an insult, saying, "She's such a busybody, always sticking her nose in where it doesn't belong." You could reframe it as, "This person must care a lot about you to tell you something she is sure you will get angry about." By reframing the situation, you can help the older driver to feel less defensive and more open to discussing a difficult topic.

ADDITIONAL EXAMPLES

Here are some more examples of the kinds of things you could say when taking a motivational interviewing approach.

EXPRESSING EMPATHY

"Mom, it sounds like trying to arrange a ride every week to church and to the grocery store when you need groceries is demanding. I think it is natural to struggle sometimes with trying to make so many changes at once. What is it like for you? Are there any situations that make it particularly difficult?"

DEVELOPING DISCREPANCIES

"So, on the one hand, you are not sticking with the driving limitations because it is hard to find a ride to the store when you want to go, but on the other hand, you worry about causing an accident or getting in legal trouble. It sounds like you really would hate to get hurt or injure someone else and would be very embarrassed if you got into legal trouble. How do you think driving when you are not allowed to affects things overall? Where does that alternate transportation plan fit in here?"

SUPPORTING SELF-EFFICACY

"I see that you have been arranging rides to get to your doctor appointments despite the hassle of making all the arrangements. It looks like you've had a lot of success making these initial changes. What's worked well for you?"

ROLLING WITH RESISTANCE

"It can be very frustrating to make all these changes, especially when you have to rely on others for rides and help. I think it's completely normal to want to go back to the way things used to be. Can I tell you about some options that I've heard worked well for others trying to make this change from driver to passenger? If you'd like, I'd be glad to help you problem solve around some of the barriers that are making these changes difficult."

This chapter has covered key points to keep in mind as you prepare to talk about change with your loved one. The next chapter will provide additional examples and practice exercises to help you gain confidence in using these techniques in your conversations. Mastering information and gaining confidence in your communication skills will prepare you to be successful in your discussions about driving fitness and safety.

CHAPTER 7

Get Talking

With your plan in place and as many bases covered as possible, it is time to sit down and start the talking. In Chapter 6, I described the theoretical basis for motivational interviewing. This chapter focuses on the *practical* side of using empathy, reflective listening, and supporting self-efficacy in your talks. I'll illustrate these skills with dialogues that show both effective and ineffective techniques.

The following conversations between a mother (Rose), and her daughter (Marge), are all based on the same set of background facts—though you'll see that the talks have dramatically different outcomes.

BACKGROUND

Rose is a 79-year-old widow. She lives alone, has limitations in her peripheral vision and far visual acuity, and she also has cataracts. She has arthritis in both knees. She has gotten a few dings when parking her car in the past year and recently had a close call with a pedestrian in a crosswalk. Her only daughter Marge is very concerned about her driving safety.

Example 1

Marge:	Mom, I don't think you should drive anymore. With your bad eyesight, you can't really see well enough to drive. I'm afraid you're going to get into an accident and get hurt, or drive into a school bus or something and hurt innocent bystanders.
Rose:	I can see fine and I've been driving longer than you've been alive. Don't worry about it.
Marge:	But I *do* worry about you. And you can't see "fine" and you know it. You haven't been driving as much as you used to, and you're so stressed-out after a drive.
Rose:	Honey, I'm 79. I don't drive as much as I used to because I don't have as much to do and the price of gas is outrageous. I'm stressed-out because everyone around here drives like a madman.
Marge:	Well, at least let's make an appointment for you to see the eye doctor to get your eyes checked. You might need a new prescription for your glasses.
Rose:	These glasses are fine, I don't need new ones. Besides, these cost me more than $200, and I want to get my money's worth out of them before buying another pair.
Marge:	Come on, Mom, you can afford a new pair. It's been four years since you've had your eyes examined. I'm calling to make the appointment. I'm due for a checkup, too, and we can get our exams done at the same time and then go out for lunch.
Rose:	Oh, all right, already. Can I watch my program in peace now?

This conversation could have gone *so* much better if Marge had planned ahead using the strategies presented in Chapter 6. Where did Marge go wrong? First, by leading off with the declaration that her mother shouldn't drive anymore, Marge has created a confrontational situation. She seems fixed on getting Rose to stop driving NOW. Rose is immediately defensive, and the conversation never recovers from this first critical mistake.

In Example 2 below, Marge has planned ahead to use an open-ended question to get the conversation started. She has reviewed the concept of reflective statements and how to use them to make sure that she understands her mother's point of view. She's had to make an effort to slow down and calm herself to get into the right mind-set (discussed in Chapter 4) before beginning the conversation. Finally, instead of viewing the goal as getting her mother to stop driving immediately, her goal is to understand what Rose thinks about driving and to explore whether Rose has thought about making a change in her driving behavior.

Example 2

		Technique used
Marge:	Mom, I noticed that you seem to have a hard time seeing things when you are driving. How's it going for you?	*open-ended question*
Rose:	Hmm. I *am* having a hard time seeing, especially things on the side of the road. It makes me nervous when I drive now.	
Marge:	It sounds like it scares you to drive when you can't see well.	*simple reflection*
Rose:	Yes, it does. I wonder if the eye doctor can do anything to help me.	

Marge:	Let's find out. I'll call to make an appointment. I'm due for a checkup, too. We can get our exams at the same time and then go out for lunch.
Rose:	That sounds good. Thanks, honey.

Did you notice that the tone of the conversation in Example 2 is dramatically different from the one in Example 1? In Example 2, the discussion is completely nonconfrontational and Marge and Rose clearly are working together to solve the issue. Using open-ended questions helps them explore what Rose is thinking. When you start the conversation this way, you avoid a confrontational or judgmental approach.

Unfortunately, conversations about driving cessation seldom go that smoothly. Example 3 shows Marge starting with the same approach, but in this illustration Rose is a little more resistant to discussing driving.

Example 3

		Technique used
Marge:	Mom, I noticed that you seem to have a hard time seeing things when you are driving. How's it going for you?	*open-ended question*
Rose:	Oh fine . . . no problems.	
Marge:	So, you don't have any problems seeing things when you are driving?	*restatement for clarification*
Rose:	Right.	

Marge: Mom, take a look at this driving
          form that I filled out Saturday after
          we drove to the beauty salon.
          According to this, you had two vision-
          related warning signs. Remember
          how hard it was for you to see
          where the lane was and the traffic
          signals? And you didn't see that
          woman in the crosswalk until
          we nearly hit her! I know you
          have always taken pride in being   *feedback about*
          such a careful driver. (pause)   *performance*
          So I was just wondering, how
          do you feel about driving?   *open-ended question*

Rose: I *have* always been proud of
          being such a careful driver.
          Do you know that I've never
          had an accident or a ticket in
          my whole life? But it does
          scare me when other drivers
          come out of nowhere and honk
          at me or I don't see pedestrians
          until the last minute. It really scares me.

Marge: Let me see if I understand you.   *summarize to check*
          On one hand you are proud to   *understanding*
          be a very careful driver and on   *double-sided reflection*
          the other you are afraid that you
          aren't seeing things well enough
          to keep driving safely. Is that right?

Rose:	Yes, that's it exactly.	
Marge:	What do you think you should do?	*encourage the person having to make the change to find her own solutions*
Rose:	I don't know. (pause) Maybe I'll get my eyes checked. My prescription might need changing.	
Marge:	I'm due for a checkup, too, and we can go together. Maybe you just need a new prescription for your glasses.	
Rose:	I hope that's all it is.	

Notice that Marge didn't get flustered or frustrated when she encountered Rose's resistance. Her agenda was to explore how Rose viewed the issue and to *understand her*. That takes enormous pressure off of Marge. Instead of trying to force a resolution, she can focus on empathically understanding her mother. Note that Marge's feedback about Rose's driving performance wasn't given in an accusatory tone, but with a "here are the facts, what can we do about them?" approach. It's important to provide feedback or information in a collaborative style—don't come off as an expert or authority. Remember that you're working *together* to solve a problem.

Example 4 shows an interaction where the mother is even more resistant and hostile. Again, however, Marge stays focused on her goal (empathic understanding) and doesn't respond in kind when Rose gets angry.

Example 4

		Technique used
Marge:	Mom, I noticed that you seem to have a hard time seeing things when you are driving. How's it going for you?	*open-ended question*
Rose:	I don't have a hard time seeing things when I'm driving. What are you talking about?	*denial*
Marge:	Mom, take a look at this driving form that I filled out Saturday after we drove to the beauty salon. According to this, you have two vision-related warning signs. Remember how hard it was for you to see where the lane was and the traffic signals? And you didn't see that woman in the crosswalk until we nearly hit her! I know you have always taken pride in being such a careful driver. (pause)	*feedback about performance*
	So I was just wondering, how do you feel about driving?	*open-ended question*
Rose:	You're spying on me and filling out forms? What the hell are you doing that for? I've never had an accident or gotten a ticket. You can drive yourself to the salon next time. That's a nice way to say	

thanks for the ride. I can't
believe you!

Marge: You are angry because it feels like
I am judging your driving. *roll with resistance*

Rose: You bet I am!

Marge: Well, that's not my intention,
Mom. This is just information
that we can discuss together.
I just want to understand what
you think about your driving safety. *open-ended question*

Rose: I think I'm a very safe driver.
As I said, I've never had an
accident or gotten a ticket.

Marge: I know . . . you've always
been a safe driver.

Rose: That's right, I have.

Marge: How would you feel if someday
you had trouble driving safely
because of vision or health
problems? *open-ended question*

Rose: Well . . . I'd probably be scared
to death I might hurt someone.
And stuck. How would I ever
go anywhere? But I *don't*
have problems!

Marge: Still, it sounds like you're saying
that it's scary to think about not
being able to drive. *restatement*

Rose:	Yes. It would kill me to be stuck at home or in a nursing home somewhere.	
Marge:	Well, you're getting a little ahead of things here. I'm not talking about being stuck at home or in a nursing home. Let's just talk about doing everything we can to make sure you can keep driving safely for as long as possible.	*shifting focus*
Rose:	That's what I want, too.	
Marge:	Do you think it might help to see your eye doctor?	
Rose:	It might. I haven't been to see her for a while. Maybe my prescription has changed.	*allow person to formulate solution*
Marge:	That's a good idea. Would you like me to make an appointment? I need an exam, too, and we could go together.	

Examples 2, 3, and 4 demonstrated ways to use the skills of reflective listening, asking open-ended questions, and rolling with resistance. Marge tried to understand her mother's perspective on driving without undue pressure or confrontation. That's the first step in the process.

ROSE'S CASE, CONTINUED

The news from the eye doctor is not good: Rose's vision is so impaired that she is no longer medically qualified to drive. The doctor tells her the news and reports her case to the DMV. She receives a letter asking her to surrender her license within 30 days. Rose is very upset, has sworn to never see this doctor again, and has threatened to report her for incompetence.

Let's see how Marge can use her communication skills to help Rose work through this distressing news.

Example 5

		Technique used
Marge:	I told you, Mom, your vision is so bad that you shouldn't be driving. I knew it.	*demeaning language*
Rose:	I hope you're happy. This is the worst day of my life.	
Marge:	Oh c'mon . . . it's not so bad. I can go grocery shopping for you and drive you around on weekends. It'll be fine—and this way you won't be a danger to anybody.	*minimizes*
Rose:	I can't believe I can't drive anymore. I feel like I've been given a prison sentence. Now I'll just wait to die.	
Marge:	Oh, Mom, don't be so melodramatic. I'll take care of everything. What should we do with your car? Do you think Richie would want it?	*acts like the expert* *takes control*

Rose:	I don't know . . . I'm just tired.
	I'm going to lie down for a while.

This may seem like an extreme example, but even the most well intentioned people can engage in behaviors that are insensitive. It may be that Marge didn't plan ahead before beginning the conversation.

Let's take a look at a more collaborative, empathic interaction.

Example 6

Marge:	Mom, how are you doing	
	after all this?	*open-ended question*
Rose:	I'm outraged at that stupid	
	doctor. I wish Dr. Feldman	
	hadn't retired; he never	
	would have done this to me.	
	I can't believe she reported me!	
Marge:	It sounds like you're angry that	
	the doctor had to report you	
	to the DMV.	*simple reflection*
Rose:	Yes. It's humiliating. Why did she	
	have to do that? I would have	
	stopped driving soon enough.	
	Now I feel like a criminal.	
Marge:	You feel embarrassed that she	
	didn't trust you enough to	
	stop driving on your own.	*simple reflection*
Rose:	Yes. Now I'm going to become	
	a shut-in who is a burden on	
	others. What kind of life is that?	

Marge:	Do you think it will be impossible to get out when you want if you can't drive?	*amplified reflection*
Rose:	Well, maybe not impossible, but awfully difficult.	
Marge:	We'll work on this challenge together, Mom. You have always managed so well before, I believe you'll be able to make the best of this, too.	*encourage self-efficacy*
Rose:	Thanks, honey. I sure hope so.	

That's a striking difference from Example 5, isn't it? I hope that all of the examples in this chapter encourage you to use an empathic and collaborative approach in your talks about driving safety, restriction, or cessation.

I encourage you to practice with a friend or family member if you're still unsure about how to do this. Ask your practice mate to think about some personal behavior they want to change. Chances are that it will be weight loss, quitting smoking, better money management or some behavior along those lines. Start off with an open-ended question, then practice using reflections, etc., until you have understood what the pros and cons of the behavior change are and how ready to change the person is. You might even want to ask him or her to complete the decision grid included in Chapter 6 so that you can practice talking about the pros and cons of a change in behavior. After some practice listening empathically and talking about sensitive topics, the process will seem less daunting.

Now that you're ready, it's up to you to start talking. Good luck!

CHAPTER 8

Resolving Dilemmas

This book gives you a road map to help you navigate the many uncertainties surrounding older drivers and safety. If you are concerned about the driving safety of yourself or a loved one, your first step is to accurately assess driving fitness and performance. Your options range from the simple worksheets included in this book, to the AAA Roadwise Review™ program, to specialized medical, vision, and professional assessments. Given the importance of driving and the consequences at stake, I encourage you to undertake the full range of assessments. The benefits of a complete assessment include your own peace of mind, the creation of hard facts on which to base decisions, a determination about whether driver retraining is a viable option, and the establishment of connections with skilled, compassionate professionals. These benefits more than offset any costs of the assessments themselves that aren't covered by Medicare or other insurance.

In Chapter 1, I described currently available assessment and retraining tools. There are also others that may be widely instituted, thanks to some promising research. We know that simply requiring in-person license renewals of drivers 85 years of age or older screens out many functionally impaired drivers and saves lives. Some states have such requirements, and more are likely to follow suit in the future. Investigators at the University of Alabama at Birmingham are hard at work conducting research to determine if simple, accurate screening assessments can feasibly be performed by state motor vehicle departments. Exciting preliminary results suggest that tests of cognitive function are able to identify drivers who are at risk for future accidents in which they are at fault. Fortunately, one of the cognitive functions that signals crash risk—processing speed—seems to be able to be improved with training. Other research advances include the potential use of driving simulators to identify or retrain at-risk drivers.

A key message of this book is that driving requires healthy functioning in three key areas: vision, thinking, and movement. Many medical conditions and certain medications affect these functions and, thus, can decrease driver safety. It is important to talk openly and often with your doctor, pharmacist, or other health professional so that any problems can be addressed early, when they are most correctable.

Above all, it's important to take the time to develop a thoughtful action plan for maintaining driver safety. In a crisis, it's very easy to respond without fully considering all options or in ways that, though well-intentioned, might be upsetting because of their tone or implications. Slow down, be patient. This is a *process* that usually takes some time. Be sure that all the steps discussed in Chapter 4 are covered, including taking care of your own needs if you are a caregiver. Also be sure to take into account the legal and regulatory realities explained in Chapter 5. In the extreme situation where you know that an older driver is clearly a safety risk but the person refuses to stop driving, you can use the sample letter as an example to follow for reporting him or her to your state's department of motor vehicles.

Of course, I hope that your situation won't be that dire and that you'll be able to solve your own driving dilemma through education, cooperation with health professionals, and productive conversations with all parties. Rely on the basics of communicating in a positive, nonconfrontational, collaborative style, as explained in Chapters 6 and 7. By embracing the spirit and techniques of motivational interviewing, and by understanding that the decision to change ultimately rests with the driver, you will be able to work *together* to resolve the driving dilemma in a way that minimizes the potential emotional damage that typically occurs in coercive approaches.

The older adult in question is—both literally and figuratively—in the driver's seat. Unless he or she is medically or legally incapable of making rational decisions, the driver is the one who has to decide to change. Your support and understanding will be a treasured resource when your loved one grapples with the decision. Drivers with diminished mental capacity present added challenges because of the illness itself and the resulting difficulties in communication. However, even in these situations the information and approaches presented here will help everyone involved move through the process as smoothly as possible.

Assistive Devices

There are many assistive devices available that can keep older drivers safe on the road. A wonderful DVD developed and produced by experts at the Gerontology Institute at the University of Massachusetts Boston illustrates what they are and how to use them. (Instructions on how to obtain a copy of the DVD are included in Appendix 3.)

To help adapt to visual challenges, consider

- A visor extender to reduce glare from the sun.

- Convex side or rearview mirrors to help eliminate blind spots.

To adapt to movement challenges, consider

- Pedal extenders to make it easier to reach the gas and brake pedals.

- Portable support handles to make it easier to get in or out of the car.

- Ceiling hand grips.

- A trash bag or silk scarf used as a seat cover to make it easier to slide in and out of the car.

- Safety belt extenders which raise the receptacle and make it easier to fasten.

- A ribbon attached to the safety belt that makes it much easier to pull over the shoulder.

- A safety belt adjuster, which positions the safety belt for easier reach.

- A safety belt pad (soft cloth or fleece) that covers a portion of the safety belt for a more comfortable fit.

- Seat cushions to raise the driver for an obstruction-free line of sight.

- A key extender, which is useful for drivers with arthritis and makes it easier to insert and turn the ignition key.

I hope this book will help you avoid the pain, confusion, and hurt feelings that have befallen less informed and less prepared families when confronted with this issue. I hope it spurs you to more open, collaborative communication that enriches and strengthens your relationships. Working together, you *can* resolve the difficult challenges posed by the driving dilemma, and you can be more prepared to face any others that may follow.

Forms to Help Assess the Situation

Warning Signs

The first form helps you to determine whether the warning signs discussed in Chapter 1 are a problem. To use the form, note if the warning sign has occurred, record the date you observed it (if possible), and estimate how often this happens (for instance, every time the person drives, sometimes, or rarely). This form can be helpful in your discussions with the driver as well as with medical or driving professionals.

Name of Driver: _____

WARNING SIGN	HOW OFTEN?	DATE OBSERVED
Has been involved in a recent auto accident (within the past five years or so)		
Recently had near misses or close calls with other cars		
Has gotten traffic tickets or police warnings recently		
Has acquired scratches, dents, and dings on the car, garage, or mailbox		
Uses the turning signal incorrectly		
Does not obey traffic signs or traffic lights		
Has trouble distinguishing the gas pedal from the brake pedal		
Does not use safety belt		
Parks incorrectly or in inappropriate areas		
Drives at inappropriate speeds (either too fast or too slow)		
Gets lost driving, even in familiar areas		
Does not pay attention to pavement markings, road signs, and traffic signals		
Responses to other cars, traffic signals and/or pedestrians are delayed		
Stops in the middle of traffic		
Rides the brake pedal		

WARNING SIGN	HOW OFTEN?	DATE OBSERVED
Displays confusion, distraction, and lack of focus on the road		
Displays anxious behavior or a decrease in confidence while driving		
Makes bad judgments. Has difficulty negotiating turns and intersections		
Has difficulty judging gaps in intersections or highway exit/entrance ramps		
Hesitates over right-of-way decisions		
Drifts into the wrong lane or onto the wrong side of the road		
Fails to notice vehicles or pedestrians on the side of the road		
Has difficulty seeing over the steering wheel		
Has trouble physically moving the steering wheel, getting in or out of the car, using mirrors, or turning to look back over his or her shoulder		
Is experiencing new or worsening medical conditions		
Takes medication that impairs driving safety		
Has to drive with a copilot		
Gets honked at or passed by other drivers		
Friends and relatives are hesitant to ride with the driver		
Other *(describe)*		

Name of person completing form: _____

This next form allows a driver to assess his or her own driving.

DRIVING SAFETY QUIZ: Assess your driving fitness by taking this quiz. Check all that apply:

	Yes ☒	
Drive	☐	I often forget to buckle my seatbelt.
	☐	I frequently get honked at by other drivers.
	☐	I have been accumulating dents and dings on my vehicle.
	☐	My family members no longer like to drive with me.
	☐	I have recently been in one or more car accidents.
	☐	I have gotten traffic tickets and/or police warnings.
	☐	Lately, I have had many "near misses."
See	☐	The glare from oncoming headlights bothers me.
	☐	It is hard for me to see at night when driving.
	☐	I have trouble seeing over the steering wheel.
	☐	I usually don't see pedestrians or other cars until they are close.
	☐	I don't see signs or lights soon enough to easily respond to them.

	Yes ☒	
Move	☐	I have trouble starting the car and/or turning the wheel.
	☐	I only rely on mirrors to back up or change lanes.
	☐	Pushing down on the gas pedal or brakes is a challenge.
	☐	I have difficulty reaching the rearview mirror.
	☐	I have trouble looking over my shoulder to look behind me.
	☐	Trying to get in and out of my vehicle is hard.
Think	☐	I often get lost while driving.
	☐	It is hard to pay attention to signs, signals, and markings.
	☐	After driving, even for a short time, I am exhausted.
	☐	My reactions are slow.
	☐	I hesitate over right-of-way decisions.

How did you do on the quiz? How many did you check for?

_____ Drive

_____ See

_____ Move

_____ Think

_____ Total?

If you checked more than one box, it is time to start talking about driving fitness with your family and doctor.

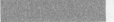

APPENDIX 2

Forms for Implementing Change

COMMUNICATE WITH YOUR DOCTOR

Doctor: _____ Today's Date:_____

Reasons why you are concerned about driving safety:

1._____

2._____

3._____

Notes to remember:

_____

_____

_____

_____

_____

Follow-up steps:

1._____

2._____

3._____

LIMITED DRIVING PLAN FORM

In order to keep driving safely for as long as possible, I agree to make the changes noted below.

Name:_____Date:_____

- I will avoid night driving.

- I will avoid driving in rain, fog, or snow.

- I will drive only on local, familiar roads.

- I will avoid left turns unless there is a traffic signal with a protected turn signal.

- I will always drive with a copilot to help me with directions.

- I will use the following assistive devices:

   ○ _____

   ○ _____

   ○ _____

If these steps are not enough to maintain safety, I want to discuss retiring from driving.

Name:_____Date:_____

Where to Find Help

Here's a list of many of the organizations that can help you. I think these first five are excellent—you may want to start with one of these.

AAA Senior Drivers (www.seniordrivers.org) This is a part of the AAA Foundation for Traffic Safety and focuses on the challenges faced by older drivers. This Web site provides safety information for seniors who are still driving as well as information for seniors who have retired from driving. Information about alternative transportation resources is available, as well as information on how to obtain the "AAA Roadwise Review" (the interactive self-assessment CD-ROM described in Chapter 1). More generally, the Foundation for Traffic Safety (www.aaafoundation.org) provides current news and updates on traffic safety, interactive tools such as fact sheets and quizzes pertaining to driving safety and presentations on safety.
AAA Foundation for Traffic Safety | 607 14th Street NW, Suite 201
Washington, DC 20005 | Tel: (202) 638-5944| Fax: (202) 638-5943

AARP (www.aarp.org) The American Association of Retired Persons is the largest nonprofit, nonpartisan membership group of adults age 50 and older. AARP provides free information, education, advocacy and services. They can give you high quality information on a broad range of topics including health, healthcare, driving safety, laws and legislation pertaining to senior adults, and more. The AARP Driver Safety Program is a refresher course for drivers 50 and older (www.aarp.org/drive).
AARP | 601 E Street NW | Washington, DC 20049
Tel: (888) OUR-AARP (888) 687-2277

The **AgeLab at the Massachusetts Institute of Technology** and **The Hartford Financial Service Group, Inc.** have teamed up to develop some excellent information about older drivers. In addition, the MIT AgeLab conducts research and offers programs in the following areas: driving and personal mobility, wellness, independent living, and caregiving. A variety of resources and services are available through the MIT AgeLab.

I think the information about dealing with dementia and driving is particularly good. To access it, go to http://www.thehartford.com/alzheimers "A Practical Guide to Alzheimer's, Dementia, and Driving." The site provides fact sheets, warning signs, and instructions on how to monitor the behavior of a driver with Alzheimer's or dementia. This guide gives tips on handling the situation and gives advice to caregivers.

The Hartford Financial Services Group | Hartford Plaza, 690 Asylum Ave. Hartford, CT 06115 | Tel: (860) 547-5000
AgeLab Massachusetts Institute of Technology
77 Massachusetts Avenue | Room E40-279 | Cambridge, MA 02139
Tel: (617) 253-0753

Association for Driver Rehabilitation Specialists (www.driver-ed.org) This organization is aimed at developing and promoting transportation modifications equipment for disabled persons or those with restricted mobility. *You can search the CDRS directory to find a Certified Driving Rehabilitation Specialist in your area. They also offer a "Fundamentals of Driver Rehabilitation" program, other training courses, and fact sheets about disabilities and driving—along with a long list of health, government, and transportation resources.

ADED | 711 S Vienna Street | Ruston, LA 71270
Tel: (318) 257-5055 or (800) 290-2344 | Fax: (318) 255-4175

ITN America (www.itnamerica.org) ITN America evolved from the Independent Transportation Network, and is an innovative approach to providing and supporting transportation services for seniors while promoting their dignity and independence. ITN provides private rather than public transportation and uses automobiles instead of vans or buses. Paid workers and volunteers provide door-to-door transportation and rides are available 24 hours a day seven days a week.

ITN America | 90 Bridge Street| Westbrook, ME 04092
Tel: (207) 854-0505 | Fax: (207) 854-1026

Aging Services and Resources

American Association of Homes and Services for the Aging (www.aahsa.org) AAHSA provides information on caregiving, transportation services and options, how to pay for services, how to plan ahead, Medicare, housing options, along with many other topics.
AAHSA | 2519 Connecticut Avenue NW | Washington, DC 20008-1520
Tel: (202) 783-2242 | Fax: (202) 783-2255 | Web site: www.info@aahsa.org

American Society on Aging (www.asaging.org) ASA offers many helpful Web seminars on promoting safety, the legal and ethical issues of aging, resources for caregivers, and more. Also available is an events calendar, links to publications on the subject of aging, and other resources. One excellent program, is the DriveWell course (www.asaging.org/drivewell/index.cfm). DriveWell is a comprehensive program providing information on how to encourage older drivers to change when and how they drive and encourage them to use alternative transportation. The program also stimulates communities to become involved in keeping older drivers safe by providing transportation options and other services to meet the needs of older adults.
American Society on Aging | 833 Market Street, Suite 511
San Francisco, CA 94103 | Tel: (415) 974-9600 or (800) 537-9728

Gerontological Society of America (www.geron.org) GSA provides researchers, educators, practitioners, and policy makers with opportunities to understand, advance, integrate, and use basic and applied research on aging to improve the quality of life of older adults. The site provides links to various journals and publications where more information may be obtained.
GSA | 1030 15th Street NW, Suite 250 | Washington DC 20005
Tel: (202) 842-1275

Loyola University Health Systems (www.luhs.org/depts/injprev/Transprt/tran3.htm) Provides safety tips for older drivers, information on where older drivers can find help, and reports on the results of research involving older drivers. Other information on health, general safety, programs offered, and transportation is also available.
Loyola University Health System | 2160 S First Ave. | Maywood, IL 60153
Tel: (708) 216-9000

National Academy on an Aging Society (www.agingsociety.org) The Academy conducts research on issues related to population aging and provides information to the public, the press, policy makers, and academic communities. Provides resources for older drivers and older workers and persons suffering from chronic and/or disabling conditions. Demographic and aging data is also accessible in reports and publications.

*The National Academy on an Aging Society is the policy institute of *The Gerontological Society of America*.

1030 15th Street NW, Suite 250 | Washington, DC 20005

Tel: (202) 408-3375 | Fax: (202) 842-1150 | Web site: www.info@agingsociety.org

National Association of Area Agencies on Aging (www.n4a.org) This organization provides general information on a broad range of topics relating to the older adult such as elder care, Medicare, and legislation. It also offers different programs for the elderly including a volunteer promotion program and an older driver safety program.

National Association of Area Agencies on Aging

1730 Rhode Island Avenue NW, Suite 1200 | Washington, DC 20036

Tel: (202) 872-0888 | Fax: (202) 872-0057

National Institute on Aging (www.niapublications.org) Part of the U.S. National Institutes of Health, NIA provides a broad range of information for older adults including the topics of men's and women's health, Alzheimer' disease, caregiving, healthy aging, planning and decision making, safety, medication and medical care, and other topics. The site provides links to related organizations, information on clinical trials, and current news and events.

National Institute on Aging | Building 31, Room 5C27

31 Center Drive, MSC 2292 | Bethesda, MD 20892

Tel: (301) 496-1752 or (800) 222-2225 | Fax: (301) 496-1072

The American Geriatrics Society (http://www.americangeriatrics.org/) Provides information on healthy aging, public policy, healthcare delivery systems, and other topics. Journals, interactive presentations, guides and handbooks are available on a variety of topics relating to the older adult.

American Geriatrics Society | The Empire State Building

350 Fifth Avenue, Suite 801 | New York, NY 10118

Tel: (212) 308-1414 | Fax: (212) 832-8646

Driver Safety Resources

Gerontology Institute, University of Massachusetts Boston (www.geront. umb.edu) Dr. Nina Silverstein and colleagues developed the DVD, *Keep*

Moving Longer: Features for Safe Driving. The 23-minute DVD shows many assistive devices and how to use them. To order, contact the Gerontology Institute. Prices: $6 single copies; $4 per copy for two-to-ten-copies; Make checks payable to the Gerontology Institute.
University of Massachusetts Boston
Gerontology Institute/*Keep Moving Longer* DVD
100 Morrissey Blvd.
Boston, MA 02125

American Association of Motor Vehicles Administrators (www.aamva.org)
An information clearinghouse with information on driver safety, driver legislation and many other topics. The Association has developed several "At-Risk Driver Programs" with one entitled "GrandDriver" which is an information and awareness campaign to educate the public about the effects of age on driving ability and to encourage drivers to make wise choices as they grow older.
AAMVA | 4301 Wilson Blvd., Suite 400 | Arlington, VA 22203
Tel: (703) 522-4200

American Driver and Traffic Safety Education Association (adtsea.iup.edu)
This organization promotes traffic safety education and provides teacher credentialing services and other educational programs. A variety of driver education resources and tools are available through this site.
ADTSEA/NSSP Highway Safety Center
Indiana University of Pennsylvania | R&P Building | Indiana, PA 15705
Tel: (724) 357-4051 or (800) 896-7703 | Fax: (724) 357-7595

Insurance Institute for Highway Safety (www.hwysafety.org) This is an independent, nonprofit, scientific and educational organization dedicated to reducing the losses—deaths, injuries, and property damage—from crashes on the nation's highways. The site provides information on driver safety, vehicle ratings, and laws and regulations.
Insurance Institute for Highway Safety | 1005 N Glebe Road, Suite 800
Arlington, VA 22201 | Tel: (703) 247-1500 | Fax: (703) 247-1588
Highway Loss Data Institute | 1005 N Glebe Road, Suite 700
Arlington, VA 22201 | Tel: (703) 247-1600 | Fax: (703) 247-1595

The Roadway Safety Foundation (www.roadwaysafety.org) Provides monthly safety tips on roadway safety, a list or program activities, and a comprehensive guide on roadway safety.

Roadway Safety Foundation | 1101 14th Street NW, Suite 750
Washington, DC 20005 | Tel: (202) 857-1200 | Fax: (202) 857-1220

Federal Agencies and Resources

Administration on Aging (www.aoa.gov) A division of the U.S. Department of
Health and Human Services. Contains information on various topics relating
to the elderly such as nutrition, housing, transportation, volunteer opportunities, etc. It also provides a news section with information on Medicare, legislation pertaining to older adults, and fact sheets. In addition, this site has
resources for caregivers and family.
Administration on Aging | Washington, DC 20201 | Tel: (202) 619-0724

Bureau of Transportation Statistics (www.bts.gov) Provides comprehensive
and current statistics on transportation costs and trends. It also supplies links to
other transportation data sources.
Bureau of Transportation Statistics | 400 7th Street SW, Room 3430
Washington, DC 20590 | Tel: (800) 853-1351

Centers for Disease Control and Prevention (www.cdc.gov/ncipc/factsheets/
older.htm) This is a direct link to the National Center for Injury Prevention
and Control's Older Adult Drivers Fact sheet, which gives information on the
occurrence of motor vehicle accidents among older adults along with the consequences of these accidents, groups at risk, risk factors, and protective factors.
National Center for Injury Prevention and Control | Mailstop K65
4770 Buford Highway NE | Atlanta, GA 30341-3724
Tel: (770) 488-1506 | Fax: (770)488-1667

Center for Transportation Analysis (cta.ornl.gov/cta) CTA is a federally
funded research center located in the Oak Ridge National Laboratory (ORNL).
They conduct research on defense transportation, highway safety, transportation systems, along with other areas of interest. CTA has generated a report
entitled "Projecting Fatalities in Crashes involving Older Drivers 2000-
2005."
National Transportation Research Center Oak Ridge National Laboratory
2360 Cherahala Boulevard | Knoxville, TN 37932
Tel: (865) 946-1349 | Fax: (865) 946-1314

ElderCare Locator (www.eldercare.gov) This site connects older adults and
caregivers to different types of senior services such as housing, transportation,

and care offered by local communities and state funded organizations. Also available are fact sheets, assessment tools, and a glossary of terms all relating to older adults. Tel: (800) 677-1116

Federal Transit Administration (www.fta.dot.gov) Part of the U.S. Dept. of Transportation, the FTA provides comprehensive information regarding transportation resources, safety, and funding. They work to improve and maintain the public transit system in our country and provide information on alternative forms of transportation.
FTA Administration's Office | 400 7th Street SW | Washington, DC 20590

FirstGov for Seniors (www.firstgov.gov/Topics/Seniors.shtml) This site provides a comprehensive list of resources for the older adult pertaining to consumer protection, jobs, education and volunteerism, federal and state agencies, health, laws and regulations, retirement, taxes, travel, and leisure.
1800 F Street NW | Washington, DC 20405
Tel: (800) FED INFO (800-333-4636)

National Eye Institute (www.nei.nih.gov) Provides public education programs on glaucoma, diabetic eye disease, and low vision which may all effect driving abilities. Also available is a clinical studies database, a public information network, and videos of public service ads.
National Eye Institute | 2020 Vision Place | Bethesda, MD 20892-3655
Tel: (301) 496-5248

National Highway Traffic Safety Administration (www.nhtsa.dot.gov/people/injury/olddrive) Printable booklets and materials are available through this site such as "Driving Safely While Aging Gracefully" and "Assessing and Counseling Older Drivers," just to name a few. Also available are resources and data, research studies, and reports to Congress, all relating to the older driver.
http://www.nhtsa.dot.gov/people/injury/olddrive/modeldriver/vol2scr.pdf This is a printable technical report on the "Model Driver Screening and Evaluation Program," which was an older driver pilot study conducted in Maryland. The report details the study methods, data, and findings.
NHTSA Headquarters | 400 Seventh Street SW | Washington, DC 20590
Tel: (888) 327-4236 or (800) 424-9153

U.S. Department of Transportation (www.fhwa.dot.gov) A direct connection to the Federal Highway Administration homepage. Provides travel and safety tips and information on how to drive in inclement weather and in traffic.

Information is also available on the different programs and funding offered by the FHWA.
Federal Highway Administration | 400 Seventh Street SW
Washington, DC 20590 | Tel: (202) 366-0660

Organizations

Alzheimer's Association (www.alz.org) Provides comprehensive information on Alzheimer's disease including what it is, the causes, warning signs, diagnosis, treatment, stages, myths, statistics, and related disorders. Also available are countless fact sheets on different topics such as driving, home safety, healthy eating, bathing, legal plans, medical care, respite care, and many more topics. The association offers resources relating to advocacy, research, and other helpful services as well.
Alzheimer's Association | 225 N Michigan Ave., Fl. 17 | Chicago, IL 60601-7633
Tel: (800) 272-3900 or (312) 335-8700 | Fax: (312) 335-1110

American Medical Association (www.ama-assn.org) Provides an extensive range of professional resources covering medical ethics, public health, legal issues, medical science, and other topics. AMA also provides links to various medical journals and has a section with current medical news and updates.
American Medical Association | 515 N State Street | Chicago, IL 60610
Toll Free: (800) 621-8335

American Public Transportation Association (www.apta.com) Provides information on the public transportation annual report and information on transportation research and statistics. Also available are lists and calendars of each mode of public transportation offered by each state.
American Public Transportation Association | 1666 K Street NW
Washington, DC 20006 | Tel: (202) 496-4800 | Fax: (202) 496-4321

American Occupational Therapy (www.aota.org) This site provides consumer information on the practice of occupational therapy and the benefits it may bring to an injured, disabled or elderly person. Also available is a "Driving and Transportation Alternative for the Older Driver" fact sheet along with resources to locate other helpful organizations and occupational therapists within your local area. This site also boasts a comprehensive online library with links to various journals, databases, and other resources containing information on occupational therapy, allied health, and other health-related areas of interest.

The American Occupational Therapy Association, Inc.
4720 Montgomery Lane | P.O. Box 31220 | Bethesda, MD 20824-1220
Tel: (301) 652-2682

Beverly Foundation (www.beverlyfoundation.org) This foundation promotes research, education, and demonstration in order to provide older adults with the ability to live independently in their community for as long as possible. Educational presentations, research reports, and information on their offered programs is available.
Beverly Foundation | 566 El Dorado St. #100 | Pasadena, CA 91101
Tel: (626) 792-2292 | Fax: (626) 792-6117

Easter Seals (www.easterseals.com) Provides information on how to make life more accessible for people who are elderly, injured, or disabled. Also available are a list of services provided by the organization such as adult day programs, medical assistance and rehabilitation, and transportation options and resources. In addition, Easter Seals provides tips on how to safeguard or adapt a house for a person whose mobility is restricted. A legislative advocacy center has also been established by Easter Seals which delivers accurate information on current news such as Medicare and other public policies.
Easter Seals | 230 West Monroe Street, Suite 1800 | Chicago, IL 60606
Tel: (312) 726-6200 or (312) 726-4258 or (800) 221-6827
Fax: (312) 726-1494

Emergency Nurses Association (www.ena.org/encare/institute/healthy_aging/default.asp) ENA provides a series of CD-ROM programs, brochures, and slide presentations all available for purchase, which cover topics such as safe medication use and falls prevention for older adults, safe driving decisions and pedestrian safety, and safe mobility.
Emergency Nurses Association Headquarters | 915 Lee Street
Des Plaines, IL 60016-6569 | Tel: (800) 900-9659

National Safety Council (www.nsc.org) NSC is dedicated to protecting life and promoting health. There are resources available on driving, falls, poison, and other potential safety hazards. Consulting services, a complete library, safety statistics, a list of upcoming events, and articles from *Safety and Health Magazine* are all available.
1121 Spring Lake Drive | Itasca, IL 60143-3201
Tel: (630) 285-1121 | Fax: (630) 285-1315

Transportation Research Board (www.trb.org) The board promotes transportation safety through research. Newsletters, articles, and publications relating to transportation needs, safety, and trends are available.

Committee on the Safe Mobility of Older Persons (www.eyes.uab.edu/safe mobility) Part of the Transportation Research Board, this committee provides countless articles, newsletters, and publications on the safe mobility of older adults.

Transportation Research Board Keck Center of the National Academies 500 Fifth Street NW | Washington, DC 20001

Transportation Resources

American Association of State Highways and Transportation Officials (safety. transportation.org) Provides a newsletter, assessment tools, and presentations all pertaining to driving safety. This organization has also developed a comprehensive guide entitled "Reducing Collisions Among Older Drivers." The guide may be accessed directly at: http://trb.org/publications/nchrp/nchrp_rpt_500v9.pdf
American Association of State Highway and Transportation Officials
444 N Capitol Street NW, Suite 249 | Washington, DC 20001
Tel: (202) 624-5800

Community Transportation Association (www.ctaa.org) Produces the *Senior Transportation* magazine which may be accessed through their site. Also available is the "Senior Transportation: Toolkit and Best Practices" comprehensive guide providing information on different types of transportation available to those in need. The site also contains a comprehensive calendar of events and has a section with current news and newly developed programs relating to transportation and services for older adults.
Community Transportation Association of America
1341 G Street NW, 10th Floor | Washington, DC 20005
Tel: (202) 628-1480 or (800) 891-0590 | Fax: (202) 737-9197

National Mobility Equipment Dealers Association (www.nmeda.org/) This organization manufactures and installs mobility equipment in vehicles for drivers and passengers with disabilities or limited mobility and provides a comprehensive list of dealers and manufacturers of mobility equipment.
NMEDA | 3327 W Bearss Ave. | Tampa, FL 33618
Tel: (800) 833-0427 or (813) 264-2697 | Fax: (813) 962-8970

Taxicab, Limousine and Paratransit Association (www.tlpa.org) A resource for locating privately owned transportation companies. A state-by-state list of independent transportation agencies is available.
Taxicab, Limousine & Paratransit Association | 3849 Farragut Avenue
Kensington, MD 20895 | Tel: (301) 946-5701 | Fax: (301) 946-4641

Internet Resources

Adaptive Driving Alliance (www.adamobility.com) A nationwide group of vehicle modification dealers who provide van conversions, hand controls, wheelchair lifts, scooter lifts, tie-downs, conversion van rentals, paratransit, and other adaptive equipment for disabled drivers and passengers or persons with restricted mobility. The alliance provides information on how to evaluate and assess a person's driving capabilities. The site also provides the names of suppliers and dealers of modified vehicles as well as links to other resources.
Adaptive Driving Alliance | 4218 W Electra Lane | Glendale, AZ 85310
Tel: (623) 434-0722 | Fax: (623) 434-1410

AgeNet (www.agenet.com) Aimed at providing solutions for better aging. Information on health, drugs, insurance, legislation, housing, care, and finances for older adults is available through this Web site.
AgeNet, Inc. | 17 Applegate Ct., Suite 200 | Madison, WI 53713
Tel: (888) 405-4242| Fax: (608) 256-3944

DriveABLE (www.driveable.com) A company associated with the University of Alberta that provides a scientifically based driving evaluation procedure to identify persons who have become unsafe to drive due to cognitive impairment. The DriveABLE Assessment is a comprehensive evaluation of driving competence for all ages. A trained professional guides the driver through a number of computer-based tests that assess mental and motor skills relevant to safe driving. If questions of competence remain, a road test has been developed to reveal errors made by drivers who are unsafe because of medical conditions, while allowing safe drivers to pass the test.

How to Care: Driving (www.howtocare.com) An elder care survival guide which provides information on caregiver support, nutrition and health, communication, and practical solutions or modifications to keep your older adult safe in their home or in their vehicle.

LA4Seniors—(www.la4seniors.com/driving.htm) This site provides information on caregiving, long-term care options, and a list of senior centers within the state of California. There is a whole section entitled "Dangerous Driving and Seniors" that provides information on the warning signs of unsafe driving, ethical and moral concerns, rehabilitation and assistive devices, where to find support, and many more topics.

Articles, Guides, Booklets, Handbooks

Alzheimer's: When Driving Becomes an Issue (www.mayoclinic.com/health/alzheimers/HO00046) An article by the Mayo Clinic that provides information on how to recognize when an older adult should no longer be behind the wheel. Measures and methods on how to keep the at-risk older driver off of the road are described in detail.

Driving Decisions Workbook (www.umtri.umich.edu/library/pdf/2000-14.pdf) This workbook produced by the University of Michigan Transportation Research Institute is a comprehensive assessment of vision, general health, cognition, mobility, and ability on the road. The workbook consists of a detailed decision tree with questions that correspond to direct feedback. At the end of the workbook are questions and answers that give advice on how to make the transition from driving to relying on other modes of transportation.
University of Michigan Transportation Research Institute
2901 Baxter Road | Ann Arbor, MI 48109-2150

Physician's Guide to Assessing and Counseling Older Drivers (www.ama-assn.org/ama/pub/category/10791.html) A ten chapter comprehensive guide created by the American Medical Association which outlines what to look for when evaluating an older driver. Patient and caregiver educational materials such as a questionnaire, evaluation form, and warning signs worksheet are available.
American Medical Association | 515 N State Street | Chicago, IL 60610
Tel: (800) 621-8335

Safe Senior Citizen Helpguide (www.helpguide.org/life) Provides general information on mental health, lifelong wellness, and elder care.
http://www.helpguide.org/life/senior_citizen_driving.htm A guide to safe senior driving. This site details risk factors and warning signs that may allow you to identify unsafe driving behaviors. Safe driving tips and driving alternatives are also available through the site.

Helpguide c/o The Center for Healthy Aging
2125 Arizona Avenue | Santa Monica, CA 90404

"When You Are Concerned" Handbook for Families and Friends (aging.state.
ny.us/caring/concerned/handbook.pdf) A 56-page printable guide produced by
the New York State Office for the Aging. Several topics are covered including
how to cope with the stress of caring for an older driver, alternative transportation
options, where to find help and support and communication and intervention
advice.
New York State Office for the Aging | 2 Empire State Plaza
Albany, NY 12223-1251 | Tel: (800) 342-9871 or (518) 474-5731
Fax: (518) 486-2225

Finding Resources in Your State

*Here's a comprehensive list of resources available by state including local driving as-
sessment and rehabilitation programs, State Offices on Aging, and state driving regulations. By contacting your state Office on Aging, you can be directed to the Area
Agency on Aging closest to your home. You can be connected directly to any Area
Agency on Aging nationwide by calling* **Eldercare Locator** *at 1-800-677-1116.*

Information about state driving regulations was adapted from Chapter 8 of the
Physician's Guide to Assessing and Counseling Older Drivers, *a product of a
cooperative agreement between The American Medical Association and The
National Highway Traffic Safety Administration (2003), written by Claire Wang,
Catherine Kosinski, Joanne Schwartzberg, and Anne Shanklin. All information
was verified and updated by my research team in 2006.*

ALABAMA

State Office on Aging

Alabama Department of Senior Services
P.O. Box 301851 | 770 Washington Avenue, Suite 470
Montgomery, AL 36130 -1851
Tel: (334) 242-5743 | Toll Free: (800) 243-5463 | Fax: (334) 242-5594

Driver Rehabilitation and Assessment Programs

Alabama Department of Rehabilitation Specialists
P. O. Box 59127 | Birmingham, AL 35259-9127
Tel: (205) 870-5999 | Fax: (205) 414-8449

Driving Concerns
79 N Miller Pt. | Eclectic, AL 36024
Tel: (334) 312-2886

Independent Living Center of Mobile
P.O. Box 8623 | Mobile, AL 36689
Tel: (251) 460-0301 | Fax: (251) 341-1267

Lakeshore Rehabilitation Facility
P.O. Box 59712 | Birmingham, AL 35259
Tel: (205) 870-5999 | Fax: (205) 879-2685

Northport Medical Center DCH Rehab - Outpatient O.T.
2700 Hospital Drive | Northport, AL 35476
Tel: (205) 333-4900 | Fax: (205) 333-4322

Phase III Mobility, Inc.
7707 Troy Highway | Pike Road, AL 36064
Tel: (334) 281-2160

The University of Alabama Spain Rehabilitation Center
1717 6th Avenue South, SRC 286 | Birmingham, AL 35233
Tel: (205) 934-4966

The Callahan Eye Foundation Hospital at the University of Alabama
Center for Low Vision Rehabilitation | 1720 University Boulevard
Birmingham, AL 35249-0009 | Tel: (205) 325-8100

University of Alabama Driving Assessment Clinic
700 S 18th St., Suite 609 | Birmingham, AL 35294-0009
Tel: (205) 325-8646 | Fax: (205) 325-8692

Alabama Driving Regulations

Driver Regulation and Licensing Agency
Alabama Department of Public Safety, Driver License Division
P.O. Box 1471 | Montgomery, AL 36102-1471
Tel: (334) 242-4239 | Web site: www.dps.state.al.us

Standard Length of license validation—4 years, in person, no vision or road test.

Age-based renewal procedures—No special requirements for age.

Reporting Procedures

Physician/medical reporting	Physician reporting is encouraged.
Immunity	Available
Legal Protection	Available
DMV follow-up	Driver notified in writing of referral. For diabetes, seizures, and convulsions, a form is sent to be completed by patient's doctor.
*Other reporting	Will accept information from courts, police, other DMVs, family members, and anyone who completes and signs the appropriate forms.
Anonymity	Not anonymous or confidential. The client may request a copy of his/her medical records by completing the necessary forms, having them notarized, and paying the proper fee for copying these records.

Role of the Medical Advisory Board—The MAB assists the Director of Public Safety with the medical aspects of driver licensing. It consists of at least 18 members, with the chairmen elected on an annual basis.

ALASKA

State Office on Aging

Alaska Commission on Aging | Department of Health and Social Services
150 Third Street, No. 103 | P.O. Box 110693 | Juneau, AK 99811-0693
Tel: (907) 465-4879 | Fax: (907) 465-4716

Driver Rehabilitation and Assessment Programs

Assistance Resources of Alaska
431 E 45th Street | Anchorage, AK 99503
Tel: (907) 562-4357 | Fax: (907) 561-4328

Blind and Visually Impaired Specialist
Alaska Division of Vocational Rehabilitation
3600 Bragaw | Anchorage AK 99508
Tel: (907) 261-8233 | Toll Free: (800) 478-4467

Care Navigators
HC-5 Box 6769 B | Palmer, AK 99645
Tel: (907) 745-4295 | Fax: (907) 745-7296

Providence Outpatient Rehabilitation Services
701 East Tutor Road | Anchorage, AK 99503
Tel: (907) 565-6300 | Fax: (907) 565-6310

University of Alaska Anchorage | Alaska Geriatric Education Center
2210 Arca Drive | Anchorage, AK 99508
Tel: (907) 264-6228 | Fax: (907) 274-4802

University of Fairbanks | Alaska Geriatric Education Center
1424 Moore Street | Fairbanks, AK 99701
Tel: (907) 456-1380 | Fax: (907) 456-1396

Work Therapy Enterprises, Inc.
1549 East Tudor Road | Anchorage, AK 99507
Tel: (907) 561-6111

Alaska Driving Regulations

Driver Licensing Agency
Alaska Department of Motor Vehicles
3300 B Fairbanks Street | Anchorage, AK 99503
Tel: (907) 269-5551 | Web site: www.state.ak.us/dmv

Standard Length of license validation—5 years, mail-in every other cycle, vision testing is required at time of in-person renewal. No written or road test required.

Age-based renewal procedures—No renewal by mail for drivers aged 69+.

Reporting Procedures

Physician/medical reporting   None. However, a licensee should self-report medical conditions that cause loss of consciousness to the DMV.

Immunity   None

Legal Protection   N/A

DMV follow-up   All medical information submitted to the DMV is reviewed by Department of Public Safety personnel.

*Other reporting   Law enforcement officers, other DMVs, and family members may submit information.

Anonymity   N/A

Role of the Medical Advisory Board—Alaska does not retain an MAB.

ARIZONA

State Office on Aging

Arizona Aging and Adult Administration | Department of Economic Security
1789 W Jefferson, No. 950A | Phoenix, AZ 85007
Tel: (602) 542-4446 | Fax: (602) 542-6575

Driver Rehabilitation and Assessment Programs

Ability Driver Rehabilitation Services, Inc.
2120 W Ina Road #105B | Tucson, AZ 85714
Tel: (520) 219-0550 | Fax: (520) 219-8881

Adaptive Driving Alliance
4218 W Electra Lane | Glendale, AZ 85310
Tel: (623) 434-0722 | Fax: (623) 434-1410

Arizona Center for the Blind and Visually Impaired
3100 East Roosevelt Street | Phoenix, AZ 85008
Tel: (602) 273-7411

ASSIST! To Independence
P.O. Box 4133 | Tuba City, AZ 86045
Tel: (928) 283-6261 | Toll Free: (888) 848-1449

DriveAble Solutions
2222 E Highland Avenue, #430 | Phoenix, AZ 85016
Tel: (602) 840-8869 | Fax: (602) 840-8947

Driving to Independence, LLC
1414 West Broadway Road, Suite 230
Tempe, AZ 85282 | Tel: (480) 449-3331 | Fax: (480) 753-9428

Good Samaritan Rehabilitation Institute
1012 E Willetta | Phoenix, AZ 85006
Tel: (602) 239-2905

Arizona Driving Regulations

Driver Licensing Agency
Arizona Department of Transportation, Motor Vehicle Division
P.O. Box 2100 | Phoenix, AZ 85001-2100
Tel: (800) 251-5866 | Web site: www.dot.state.az.us/mvd/mvd.htm

Standard Length of license validation—12 years until age 65, then 5 years.
Vision testing is required at time of renewal; however, no road test is
required unless recommended by Medical Review Program.

Age-based renewal procedures—At age 65 with vision test, reduction of
cycle to 5 years. No renewal by mail after age 70.

Reporting Procedures

Physician/medical reporting	Yes (not specified)
Immunity	Available
Legal Protection	Reporting immunity is granted.
DMV follow-up	The DMV follows physician recommendations.
*Other reporting	Will accept information from courts, police, other DMVs, family members, and other sources.
Anonymity	Available

Role of the Medical Advisory Board—The Medical Review Program staff reviews reports to determine if a licensee requires a reexamination of driving skills, written testing, or medical/psychological evaluation.

Arizona Department of Transportation | Medical Review Program Mail Drop 818Z

P.O. Box 2100 | Phoenix, AZ 85001 | Tel: (623) 925-5795 | Fax: (623) 925-9323

ARKANSAS

State Office on Aging

Arkansas Division of Aging and Adult Services
Department of Human Services
P.O. Box 1437 | 700 Main Street, 5th Floor, S530
Little Rock, AR 72203-1437 | Tel: (501) 682-2441 | Fax: (501) 682-8155

Driver Rehabilitation and Assessment Programs

Arkansas Rehabilitation Services
1616 Brookwood Drive | P.O. Box 3781
Little Rock, AR 72203 | Tel: (501) 296-1669 | Fax: (501) 296-1655

Hot Springs Rehabilitation Center
Tel: (501) 624-4411 | Fax: (501) 624-0019

Increasing Capabilities Access Network (ICAN)
Tel: (501) 666-8868 | Toll Free: (800) 828-2799 | Fax: (501) 666-5319

Lions World Services for the Blind Vision Rehabilitation Services
2811 Fair Park Boulevard | Little Rock, AR 72204
Tel: (501) 664-7100 | Toll Free: (800) 248-0734 | Fax: (501) 664-2743

University of Arkansas for Medical Sciences - University Rehab
4301 W Markham St. | Little Rock, AR 72205
Tel: (501) 686-8000 | Toll Free: (800) 942-8267

Arkansas Driving Regulations

Driver Licensing Agency
Arkansas Office of Motor Vehicles
P.O. Box 31553 | Little Rock, AR 72203
Tel: (507) 682-1631 | Web site: www.state.ar.us/dfa/odd/motor_vehicle.html

Standard Length of license validation—4 years, renewal options and conditions in person, by mail only if out of state. Vision testing is required at time of renewal, however no written or road test is required.

Age-based renewal procedures—None

Reporting Procedures

Physician/medical reporting	Physician reporting is encouraged.
Immunity	None
Legal protection	None
DMV follow-up	Medical information is reviewed by the director of Driver Control. An appointment is scheduled within 2 weeks of receipt. At that time, a medical form is given to the licensee for completion by a physician. If the medical exam is favorable, a road test is given.
*Other reporting	Will accept information from courts, police, other DMVs, and family members.
Anonymity	N/A

Role of the Medical Advisory Board—Arkansas does not have a medical advisory board. However, unsafe drivers may be referred to Driver Control. Arkansas Driver Control | Hearing Officer Room 1070 1910 West 7th | Little Rock, AR 72203 | Tel: (501) 682-1631

CALIFORNIA

State Office on Aging

California Department of Aging
1300 National Drive, #200 | Sacramento, CA 95834
Tel: (916) 419-7500 | Fax: (916) 928-2268

Driver Rehabilitation and Assessment Programs

Adaptive Driving Program
P.O. Box 641 | Montebello, CA 90640-0641
Tel: (323) 855-1502 | Fax: (323) 726-8402

Adaptive Driver Program of Citrus Heights
6976 Pollen Way | Citrus Heights, CA 95610
Tel: (916) 722-8718 | Fax: (916) 722-8718

Adaptive Driving Services
616 Hobart Terrace | Santa Clara, CA 95051
Tel: (408) 984-7949 | Fax: (408) 984-7949

Adaptive Driving Systems, Inc.
7959 Deering Avenue | Canoga, Park CA 91304 | Tel: (818) 251-9876

Apex Driving School Mobility Training Division
850 Clement St., Suite 103 | San Francisco, CA 94118
Tel: (415) 221-7025

California Department of Rehabilitation Mobility Evaluation Program
9720 S Norwalk Blvd. | Santa Fe Springs, CA 90670
Tel: (562) 906-4972 | Fax: (562) 941-8719

Casa Colina Hospital for Rehabilitation Medicine
255 East Bonita Avenue | Ponoma, CA 91767 | Tel: (909) 593-7521

Central Coast Driver's Safety Evaluation
1128 Iris Street | San Luis Obispo, CA 93401 | Tel: (805) 541-5543

Creative Mobility
320 Civic Center Drive | National City, CA 91950 | Tel: (619) 474-4072

Kaweah Delta Rehabilitation Hospital
840 S Akers Rd. | Visalia, CA 93277
Tel: (559) 624-3903 | Fax: (559) 624-3779

La Palma Hospital Driving Program - Occupational Therapy
7901 Walker Street | La Palma, CA 90623
Tel: (714) 670-6000 | Fax: (714) 670-6263

Loma Linda University Medical Center Physical Medicine and
Rehabilitation
Disabled Driving Program | Tel: (909) 558-6144

Long Beach Veterans Affairs Medical Center - Driver Rehabilitation
5901 East 7th Street, #117 | Long Beach, CA 90822
Tel: (562) 826-5618 | Fax: (562) 826-8191

Nor Cal Mobility, Inc.
1300 Nord Avenue | Chico, CA 95926 | Tel: (530) 893-1111

Northridge Hospital Medical Center Driver Prep Program
18300 Roscoe Blvd., 4th Fl. – Occupational Therapy
Northridge, CA 91328 | Tel: (818) 885-5460

On the Road, Again
9590 Chesapeake Dr. Ste. 122 | San Diego, CA 92123
Tel: (858) 278-1142 | Fax: (858) 278-1115

Rancho Los Amigos National Rehabilitation Center
7601 E Imperial Hwy. | Bldg. 900 Annex B | Downey, CA 90266
Tel: (562) 401-7081 | Fax: (562) 401-6167

SCVMC/Therapy Services Adaptive Training Evaluation Program
751 S Bascom Avenue | San Jose, CA 95128
Tel: (408) 885-5613 | Fax: (408) 885-4844

Sharp Memorial Hospital Rehabilitation Center Adaptive Driving
Program
2999 Health Center Drive | San Diego, CA 92123 | Tel: (619) 541-3328

State of California Department of Rehabilitation Services
Mobility Evaluation Program |9720 Norwalk Blvd.
Santa Fe Springs, CA 90670
Tel: (562) 906-4972 | Fax: (562) 941-8719

Tri-City Medical Center
4002 Vista Way | Oceanside, CA 92056 | Tel: (760) 940-7866

University of California, Irvine SeniorHealth Center, Pavilion IV
Health Assessment Program for Seniors - HAPS
101 UCI Medical Center Drive | Orange, CA 92868

California Driving Regulations

Driver Licensing Agency
California Department of Motor Vehicles
2415 First Avenue, Mail Station C152 | Sacramento, CA 95818-2698
Tel: (916) 657-6550 | Web site: www.dmv.ca.gov

Standard Length of license validation—5 years. Renewal options and conditions are in person or (if applicant qualifies) mail renewal for no more than 2 license terms in sequence. Vision and written test is required at in-person renewal. Road test is required only if there is significant evidence of driving impairment.

Age-based renewal procedures—No renewal by mail at age 70 and older

Reporting Procedures

Physician/medical reporting	Physicians are required to report all patients diagnosed with "disorders characterized by lapses of consciousness." The law specifies that this definition includes Alzheimer's disease "and those related disorders that are severe enough to be likely to impair a person's ability to operate a motor vehicle." Physicians are not required to report unsafe drivers. However, they are authorized to report, given their good faith judgment, that it is in the public's interest.
Immunity	Yes, if the condition is required to be reported. (A physician who has failed to report such a patient may be held liable for damages.) If the condition is not required to be reported, there is no immunity from liability.
Legal protection	Only if the condition is required by law to be reported.
DMV follow-up	The medical information obtained from the physician is reviewed by DMV hearing officers within the Driver Safety Branch. The driver is reexamined; at the conclusion of the process, the DMV may take no action, impose restrictions, limit license term, order periodic reexaminations, or suspend or revoke the driver's license.

*Other reporting	The DMV will accept information from the driver him or herself, courts, police, other DMVs, family members, and virtually any other source.
Anonymity	If so requested, the name of the reporter will not be divulged (unless a court order mandates disclosure).

Role of the Medical Advisory Board—The MAB gathers specialists for panels on special driving related topics (e.g., vision). These panels develop policy recommendations for the DMV regarding drivers with a particular type of impairment. No recommendations are made regarding individuals as such.
Post Licensing Policy | California Department of Motor Vehicles
2415 First Avenue, Mail Station C163 | Sacramento, CA 95818-2698
Tel: (916) 657-5691

COLORADO

State Office on Aging

Colorado Division of Aging and Adult Services
Department of Human Services | 1575 Sherman Street, Ground Floor
Denver, CO 80203-1714 | Tel: (303) 866-2636 | Fax: (303) 866-2696

Driver Rehabilitation and Assessment Programs

Center for Neurorehabilitation Services
1045 Robertson St. | Ft. Collins, CO 80524
Tel: (970) 493-6667 | Fax: (970) 493-8016

Capron Institute of Rehabilitation - Occupational Therapy
2215 North Cascade Avenue | P.O. Box 7021
Colorado Springs, CO 80933 | Tel: (719) 630-5200

Cheyenne Mountain Rehabilitation - Occupational Therapy
660 Southpoint Court, Suite 100 | Colorado Springs, CO 80906
Toll Free: (800) 568-5957

Colorado Center for the Blind
1830 South Acoma Street | Denver, CO 80223
Tel: (303) 778-1522 | Toll free: (800) 401-4632

Colorado Rehabilitation Services - Colorado Department of Human Services
110 16th Street | Denver, CO 80203 | Tel: (303) 620-2152

Craig Hospital Adaptive Driving Program
3425 South Clarkson Street | Englewood, CO 80110
Tel: (303) 789-8218 | Fax: (303) 721-0526

MasterDrive
3280 E Woodman Rd., Suite 100 | Colorado Springs, CO 80918
Tel: (719) 260-0999 | Fax: (719) 260-9676
15659 East Hinsdale Drive | Englewood, CO 80111
Tel: (303) 627-4447 | Fax: (303) 721-0526

Memorial Hospital Senior Clinic
Printers Park Medical Plaza | 175 S Union, Suite 300
Colorado Springs, CO | Tel: (719) 365-6363

Spalding Rehabilitation Hospital
900 Potomac Street |Aurora, CO 80011
Tel: (303) 363-5163 | Fax: (303) 363-5634

Swedish Medical Center - Rehabilitation Services
7001 South Willow Street | Englewood, CO 80112 | Tel: (720) 428-7484

Colorado Driving Regulations

Driver Licensing Agency
Colorado Department of Motor Vehicles | Driver License Administration
1881 Pierce Street, Room 136 | Lakewood, CO 80214
Tel: (303) 205-5664 | Web site: www.mv.state.co.us/mv.html

Standard Length of license validation—10 years. Renewal options and conditions: If eligible, mail-in every other cycle. Vision testing is required at time of renewal. Written test is required only if point accumulation results in suspension. Road test is not required unless condition has developed since last renewal that warrants road test.

Age-based license procedures—At age 61, renewal period is reduced to every 5 years and no renewal by mail.

Reporting Procedures

Physician/medical reporting	Drivers should self-report medical conditions that may cause a lapse of consciousness, seizures, etc. Physicians are encouraged but not required to report patients who have a medical condition that may affect their ability to safely operate a motor vehicle.
Immunity	N/A
Legal protection	No civil or criminal action may be brought against a physician or optometrist licensed to practice in Colorado for providing a written medical or optometric opinion.
DMV follow-up	The driver is notified in writing of the referral and undergoes a reexamination. Medical clearance may be required from a physician, and restrictions may be added to the license.
*Other reporting	Will accept information from courts, police, other DMVs, and family members.

Role of Medical Advisory Board—Colorado does not currently retain a medical advisory board. *Unless the customer is blind in one eye, individual eye acuity is not normally tested nor is there an individual eye minimum acuity requirement. The DMV is concerned with the acuity of both eyes together. **Based on discussions with ophthalmologists and optometrists, the DMV does not currently test peripheral vision or color vision as accommodations can be made for these deficiencies. However, testing is performed for phoria.

CONNECTICUT

State Office on Aging

Connecticut Bureau of Aging Community & Social Work Services
Department of Social Services
25 Sigourney Street | Hartford, CT 06106
Tel: (860) 424-5277 | Fax: (860) 424-5301

Driver Rehabilitation and Assessment Programs

Bridgeport Hospital Ahlbin Centers for Rehabilitation Medicine
226 Mill Hill Ave. | Bridgeport, CT 06610
Tel: (203) 366-7551 | Fax: (203) 336-5465
2600 Post Rd. | Fairfield, CT 06490
Tel: (203) 259-7117 | Fax: (203) 259-1071
4 Corporate Dr. | Shelton, CT 06484
Tel: (203) 925-4201
3585 Main St. | Stratford, CT 06614
Tel: (203) 380-4672

Bristol Hospital Rehab Dynamics
975 Farmington Ave. | Bristol, CT 06010 | Tel: (860) 589-3587

Center for Adaptive Technology
SCSU, Engelman Hall, Rm. 5 | New Haven, CT 06515
Tel: (203) 392-5799 | Fax: (203) 392-5796

Connecticut Department of Motor Vehicles Handicapped Driver
60 State Street | Wethersfield, CT 06161 | Tel: (860) 263-5086

Department of Rehabilitation and Sports Medicine
Medical Arts & Research Building at UConn Health Center
263 Farmington Avenue | Farmington, CT 06030-5153
Tel: (860) 679-3233

Easter Seals Mobility Center
158 State Street | Meriden, CT 06450
Tel: (203) 237-7835 | Fax: (203) 237-9187
Web site: www.ct.easterseals.com

Gaylord Hospital Driver Assessment/Rehabilitation Program
P.O. Box 400 Gaylord Farm Rd. | Wallingford, CT 06492
Tel: (203) 284-2820 | Fax: (203) 284-2876

Lions Low Vision Centers
33 Highland St. | New Britain, CT 06050
Tel: (860) 832-9601 | Toll Free: (800) 676-5715 | Fax: (860) 832-9604
710 Brewster St. | Bridgeport, CT 06605 | Toll Free: (800) 676-5715

McLean Outpatient Rehabilitation
75 Great Pond Road | Simsbury, CT 06070
Tel: (860) 658-3998 | Fax: (860) 658-3764
Web site: www.mcleancare.org

Adler Geriatric Assessment Center - The Driving Programs at Yale
Yale-New Haven Hospital, Tompkins Building
789 Howard Avenue | New Haven, CT 06536-0805 | Tel: (203) 688-3344

Connecticut Driving Regulations

Driver Licensing Agency
Connecticut Department of Motor Vehicles
60 State Street | Wethersfield, CT 06161-2510
Tel: (860) 263-5700 or (860) 842-8222 | Web site: www.dmvct.org

Standard Length of license validation—6 years. One can renew in person at DMV, mobile unit scheduled locations, satellite offices, license renewal centers, and authorized AAA offices. There is no vision or written test. Road test is only required for new applicants and for these applicants whose license has been expired for two or more years.

Age-based renewal procedures—Applicants age 65+ may renew for 2 years or 6 years. Applicants age 65+ may renew by mail only upon submission of a written application showing hardship which shall include, but is not limited to, distance of applicant's residence from DMV renewal facility.

Reporting Procedures

Physician/medical reporting	Sec 14–46 states that a "physician may report to the DMV in writing the name, age, and address of any person diagnosed by him to have any chronic health problem which in the physician's judgment will significantly affect the person's ability to safely operate a motor vehicle."
Immunity	No civil action may be brought against the commissioner, the department or any of its employees, the board or any if its members, or any physician for providing any reports, records, examinations, opinions, or recommendations.

	Any person acting in good faith shall be immune from liability.
Legal protection	Only the laws regarding immunity apply.
DMV follow-up	The driver is notified in writing of his/her referral to the MAB. If the MAB requires additional information for review in order to make a recommendation, the driver is requested to file the additional medical information.

*Other reporting State regulations require "reliable information" to be on file for the DMV to initiate a medical review case. This includes a written, signed report from any person in the medical/law enforcement profession, or a third party report on the DMV affidavit which requires signing in the presence of a notary public.

Anonymity All information on file in a medical review case is classified as "confidential." However, it is subject to release to the person or his/her representative upon written authorization from the person to release the data.

Role of the Medical Advisory Board—The MAB must be comprised of 8 specialties (general medicine or surgery, internal medicine, cardiovascular medicine, neurology or neurological surgery, ophthalmology, orthopedic surgery, psychiatry, optometry). The MAB advises the commissioner on health standards relating to safe operation of motor vehicles; recommends procedures and guidelines for licensing individuals with impaired health; assists in developing medically acceptable standardized report forms; recommends training courses for motor vehicle examiners on medical aspects of operator licensure; undertakes any programs/activities the commissioner may request relating to medical aspects of motor vehicle operator licensure; makes recommendations and offers advice on individual health problem cases; and establishes guidelines for dealing with such individual cases.

Connecticut Department of Motor Vehicles | Medical Review Division
60 State Street | Wethersfield, CT 06161-2510
Tel: (860) 263-5223 | Fax: (860) 263-5774

DELAWARE

State Office on Aging

Delaware Division of Services for Aging and Adults with Physical
Disabilities
Department of Health and Social Services
1901 North DuPont Highway | New Castle, DE 19720
Tel: (302) 255-9390 | Fax: (302) 255-4445

Driver Rehabilitation and Assessment Programs

Bayhealth Medical Center
Milford Memorial Hospital Therapy Services:
Tel: (302) 430-5706
Kent General Hospital Physical Therapy Inpatient Services:
Tel: (302) 744-6847
Kent General Hospital Physical Therapy Outpatient Services:
Tel: (302) 744-7095

Center for Rehabilitation at Wilmington Hospital-Christiana Care
501 West 14th Street | Wilmington, DE 19801 | Tel: (302) 428-6600

Delaware Curative
North Wilmington Center | Tel: (302) 529-7750
Middletown Center | Tel: (302) 376-7670
Wilmington Center | Tel: (302) 656-5226
Newark Center | Tel: (302) 738-3110
Bear Center | Tel: (302) 836-5670
Dover Center | Tel: (302) 744-9691

Division for the Visually Impaired - Delaware Health and Social
Services
Health and Social Services Campus, Holloway Campus, Biggs Building
1901 North DuPont Highway | New Castle, DE 19720-1199
Tel: (302) 577-4730

Easter Seals Outpatient Rehabilitation Therapies
61 Corporate Circle | New Castle, DE 19720
Tel: (302) 324-4444 | Toll Free: (800) 677-3800 | Fax: (302) 324-4441

Moss Rehabilitation
18 Stearrett Drive | Newark, DE 19702 | Tel: (305) 452-0812

St. Francis Hospital Physical Medicine Rehabilitation
Clayton Building 6th Floor | 7th & Clayton Streets
Wilmington, DE 19805 | Tel: (302) 421-4697 | Fax: (302) 421-4698

Delaware Driving Regulations

Driver Licensing Agency
Delaware Division of Motor Vehicles
P.O. Box 698 | Dover, DE 19903 | Tel: (302) 744-2500 | Web site:
www.dmv.de.gov/

Standard Length of license validation—5 years, in person only. Vision test
is required, however no written or road test.

Age-based renewal procedures—None

Reporting Procedures

Physician/medical reporting	Physicians should report patients subject to "losses of consciousness due to disease of the central nervous system." Failure to do so is punishable by a fine of $5.00 to $50.00.
Immunity	Available
Legal protection	N/A
DMV *follow up*	The driver is notified in writing of the referral and his/her license is suspended until further examination.
*Other reporting	The DMV will accept information from courts, other DMVs, police, and family members.
Anonymity	The DMV protects the identity of the reporter.

Role of the Medical Advisory Board—If the DMV receives conflicting or
questionable medical reports, the reports are sent to the MAB. The MAB
determines whether the individual is medically safe to operate a motor
vehicle.

Delaware Health and Social Services
1901 N DuPont Highway | Main Building | New Castle, DE 19720
Tel: (302) 255-9040 or (302) 744-4700 | Fax: (302) 255-4429

DISTRICT OF COLUMBIA

State Office on Aging

District of Columbia Office on Aging
One Judiciary Square | 441 4th Street, NW, 9th Floor
Washington, DC 20001 | Tel: (202) 724-5622 | Fax: (202) 724-4979

Driver Rehabilitation and Assessment Programs

Georgetown University Hospital Physical and Rehabilitation Medicine
Room CG-12, Ground Floor, Bles Building |3800 Reservoir Road, NW
Washington, DC 20007 | Tel: (202) 444-4180 | Fax: (202) 444-5333

Howard University Hospital - Geriatrics
Towers Building, Suite 5000 | 2041 Georgia Avenue, NW 20060
Tel: (202) 865-3397
Department of Physical Medicine and Rehabilitation
Tel: (202) 865-1411 | Fax: (202) 865-4724

Department of Veterans Affairs Prosthetic & Sensory Aids Services
Mailing Code 117C | Washington, DC 20420 | Tel: (202) 535-7293

Providence Hospital Rehabilitation Services
1150 Varnum St. NE | Washington, DC 20017 | Tel: (202) 269-7567

National Rehabilitation Hospital - Occupational Therapy Department
102 Irving St. NW | Washington, DC 20010
Tel: (202) 877-1705 | Fax: (202) 232-1571

The NRH Driver Training Program
102 Irving Street NW | First floor, outpatient gym
Washington, DC 20010 | Tel: (202) 877-1620

Sibley Memorial Hospital Rehabilitation Medicine
5255 Loughboro Road NW | Washington DC 20016
Tel: (202) 364-7665

The George Washington University Hospital
Rehabilitation Center | 2131 K Street #620 | Washington DC 20037
Tel: (202) 715-5655
Senior Advantage Program
Tel: (202) 715-4263

Veteran Affairs Medical Center - Physical Medicine and Rehabilitation
50 Irving St. NW | Washington, DC 20422 | Tel: (202) 745-8000

Walter Reed Army Medical Center - Physical Medicine and Rehabilitation
Building 2, Room 3J | Washington DC 20307 | Tel: (202) 782-6369/3045

Washington Hospital Center - Physical Medicine and Rehabilitation
110 Irving Street, NW, GB-1 | Washington, DC 20010 |Tel: (202) 877-3627

District of Columbia Driving Regulations

Driver Licensing Agency
District of Columbia Department of Motor Vehicles
3301 C Street NW | Washington, DC 20001
Tel: (202) 727-5000 | Web site: www.dmv.dc.gov

Standard Length of license validation—5 years, renewal options and
conditions are drivers with a clear driver record and no medical requirements can now renew their license on-line. Vision and written tests are
required, however, drivers are allowed a 6-month grace period. Licensees
with physical disabilities may require a road test at the time of renewal.
Also, senior citizens may be required to take the road test on an observa-
tional basis.

Age-based renewal procedures—At age 70, the licensee must submit a letter
from his/her physician stating that the licensee is medically fit to drive
based on vision and physical and mental capabilities. At age 75 and older,
the licensee has required written and road tests.

Reporting Procedures
Physician/medical reporting	Permitted but not required
Immunity	None
Legal protection	None
DMV follow-up	N/A

Other reporting   Any concerned citizen may report.

Anonymity   Reporters are allowed to remain
                           anonymous.

Role of the Medical Advisory Board—Washington, DC, does not have a
medical advisory board.

FLORIDA

State Office on Aging

Florida Department of Elder Affairs
4040 Esplanade Way, Suite 315 | Tallahassee, FL 32399
Tel: (850) 414-2000 | Fax: (850) 414-2004

Driver Rehabilitation and Assessment Programs

Adaptive Mobility Services, Inc.
1000 Delaney Ave. | Orlando, FL 32806
Tel: (407) 426-8020 | Fax: (407) 426-8690
Web site: www.adaptivemobility.com

Advance Driving Skills Institute
2778 Countryside Blvd. #3 | Clearwater, FL 33071 | Tel: (727) 669-8308

Advanced Driver Rehabilitation, Inc.
1031 Ives Dairy Road, Suite 228 | North Miami Beach, FL 33179
Tel: (305) 770-0747 | Fax: (305) 770-0269

Advanced Driving Systems, Inc.
662 Capitol Circle NE | Tallahassee, FL 32301 | Tel: (850) 671-2300

BMC Family Health Center - Occupational Therapy Department
780 94th Ave. N, Suite 108 | St. Petersburg, FL 33702
Tel: (727) 579-8077 | Fax: (727) 577-7594

Brooks Rehabilitation
3901 University Blvd. S | Jacksonville, FL 32216
Tel: (904) 858-7242 | Fax: (904) 858-7255
Web site: www.brookshealth.org

Buddy's Sunset Mobility Center
8415 SW 129 Terrace | Miami, FL 33156 | Tel: (305) 234-0071

Department of Veterans Affairs
1849 NW 126 Way | Coral Springs, FL 33071
10311 SE Jupiter Narrows Drive | Hobe Sound, FL 33455
Tel: (561) 422-7765 | Fax: (561) 422-8288

Driver Rehabilitation Services, Inc.
9315 Hunters Park Way | Tampa, FL 33647
Tel: (800) 738-9967 | Fax: (866) 738-9967

Easter Seals Society of Southwest Florida - Driver Training
350 Braden Avenue | Sarasota, FL 34243 | Tel: (813) 355-7637

Gulf Shore Rehabilitation, Inc.
2709 Swamp Cabbage Ct., Suite 107 | Fort Myers, FL 33901
Tel: (239) 277-7997 | Fax: (239) 936-7820
Web site: www.gulfshorerehab.com

Handicapped Drive Services
5675 University Blvd. West | Jacksonville, FL 32216 | Tel: (904) 281-0111

HEALTHSOUTH Rehabilitation of Sarasota
3251 Proctor Road | Sarasota, FL 34231 | Tel: (941) 921-8672

James A. Haley Veteran Affairs Hospital - Corrective Therapy
13000 Bruce B. Downs Blvd. | Tampa, FL 33612 | Tel: (813) 972-2000

Memorial Rehabilitation Outpatient Center - Occupational Therapy
3901 University Blvd. South | Jacksonville, FL 32216
Tel: (904) 858-7242 | Fax: (904) 858-7240

Ocean Conversion & Mobility
750 East Sample Road Bldg. 8/#7 | Pompano Beach, FL 33064
Tel: (954) 942-6033 | Fax: (954) 942-6240

Pinecrest Rehabilitation Hospital
5360 Lincoln Blvd. | Delray Beach, FL 33484 | Tel: (561) 495-3634

Rehabilitation Institute of Sarasota - Occupational Therapy
3251 Proctor Road | Sarasota, FL 34231
Tel: (813) 921-8684 | Fax: (813) 921-8690

Safe-Tech Solutions
190 Wilson Blvd. North | Naples, FL 34120 | Tel: (914) 352-8771

Shands Rehab Hospital
4101 NW 89th Blvd. | Gainesville, FL 32606
Tel: (352) 265-5487 | Fax: (352) 265-5431

Sunrise Rehabilitation Center - Occupational Therapy
4399 Nob Hill Road | Sunrise, FL 33351 | Tel: (517) 667-1366

Tampa General Rehabilitation Center Driving Program
P.O. Box 1289 | Tampa, FL 33601 | Tel: (813) 251-7707

University of Florida College of Health Professions
National Older Driver Research and Training Center
P.O. Box 100164 | Gainesville, FL 32610
Gainesville Tel: (352) 392-8850 | (352) 273-6043
Ocala Tel: (352) 629-3015

UpReach Pavillion - Occupational Therapy
8900 Northwest 39 Avenue | Gainesville, FL 32606 | Tel: (904) 375-4129

Veteran Affairs Medical Center - Physical Medicine and Rehabilitation
1201 Northwest 16 Street | Miami, FL 33125
Tel: (305) 324-3198 | Fax: (305) 324-3385

West Florida Rehabilitation Institute - Occupational Therapy
P.O. Box 18900 | 8391 North Davis Highway | Pensacola, FL 32523
Tel: (850) 494-6167 | Fax: (850) 494-4881

Florida Driving Regulations

Driver Licensing Agency
Florida Department of Highway Safety and Motor Vehicles
Neil Kirkman Building | 2900 Apalachee Parkway
Tallahassee, FL 32399-0500
Tel: (850) 922-9000 | Web site: www.hsmv.state.fl.us.html/dlnew.html

Standard Length of license validation—4–6 years, depending on driving history. Renewal options and conditions are in person every 3rd cycle. Vision testing will be required at in-person renewal. A written test may be required based on driving history and/or observation of physical or mental impairments. A road test may be required based on observation of physical or mental impairments

Age-based renewal procedures—Effective January 2004, vision testing is required at each renewal for drivers over the age of 79.

Reporting Procedures

Physician/medical reporting	Any physician, person or agency having knowledge of a licensed driver's or applicant's mental or physical disability to drive may report the person to the Department of Highway Safety and Motor Vehicles (DHSMV). Forms are available on the DHSMV Web site, as well as at local driver license offices. The Division of Driver Licenses' (DDL) Medical Review Section provides other forms as the situation requires.
Immunity	N/A
Legal protection	The law provides that no report shall be used as evidence in any civil or criminal trial or in any court proceeding.
DMV follow-up	The DHSMV investigates, sanctions actions if needed, and notifies the driver in writing.
*Other reporting	The law authorizes any person, physician, or agency to report.
Anonymity	Available

Role of the Medical Advisory Board—The MAB advises the DHSMV on medical criteria and vision standards and makes recommendations on mental and physical qualifications of individual drivers.

DHSMV/DDL/Driver Improvement Medical Section
2900 Apalachee Parkway | Tallahassee, FL 32399-0570
Tel: (850) 488-8982 | Fax: (850) 921-6147

GEORGIA

State Office on Aging

Georgia Division for Aging Services
2 Peachtree St. NW 9th Floor | Atlanta, GA 30303
Tel: (404) 657-5258 | Fax: (404) 657-5285

Driver Rehabilitation and Assessment Programs

Atlanta Veteran Affairs Medical Center
Rehabilitation Medicine – Occupational Therapy
1670 Clarmont Road | Decatur, GA 30033 | Tel: (404) 321-6111

Candler Center for Rehabilitation
5353 Reynolds Street | Savannah, GA 31405
Tel: (912) 819-6176 | Fax: (912) 819-8829

Dekalb Medical Center
2701 N Decatur Rd. | Decatur, GA 30033
Tel: (404) 501-5841 | Fax: (404) 501-5498
Web site: www.dekalbmedicalcenter.org
417 Mimosa Driver | Decatur, GA 30030
Tel: (404) 501-7169 | Fax: (404) 501-7186

Emory Center for Rehabilitation Medicine - Occupational Therapy
248 Ribbon Leaf View | Suwanee, GA 300024
Tel: (404) 712-5527 | Fax: (404) 712-5974

Freedom & Mobility – Driver Evaluation & Training
1651 Canton Rd. | Marietta, GA 30066 | Tel: (770) 514-9957

Gwinnett Medical Center - Glancy Rehabilitation Center Outpatient
Program
3215 McClure Bridge Road | Duluth, GA 30096 | Tel: (678)584-6750

Medical College of Georgia Medical Center - Rehabilitation Services
1120 15th Street | 6th Floor West | Augusta, GA 30912
Tel: (706) 721-2481 | Fax: (706) 721-8168

Monaco's Therapy on Wheels
1225 Walton Way | Augusta, GA 30901
Tel: (706) 650-5501 | Fax: (706) 266-5502
Web site: www.therapyonwheels.com

Palmyra Rehabilitation Center
2000 Old Dominion Road | Albany, GA 31702
Tel: (912) 434-2497 | Fax: (912) 434-2596

Resource Builders, LLC
1405 Glendale Road | Marietta, GA 45750 | Tel: (740) 373-1809

Roosevelt Warm Springs Institute for Rehabilitation Driver Education
Services
P.O. Box 1000 | Warm Springs, GA 31830
Tel: (706) 655-5075 | Fax: (706) 655-5567

Shepherd Center
2020 Peachtree Rd. NW | Atlanta, GA 30309
Tel: (404) 350-7798 | Fax: (404) 350-7356

The Medical Center of Central Georgia - Golden Opportunities
3797 Northside Dr. | Macon, GA 31210
Tel: (478) 757-7817

The University of Georgia College of Public Health - Institute of Gerontology
255 E. Hancock Avenue | Athens, GA 30602-5775 | Tel: (706) 425-3222

Walton Rehabilitation Hospital
1355 Independence Drive | Augusta, GA 30901-1037
Tel: (706) 724-7746 | Toll Free: (866) 492-5866

Georgia Driving Regulations

Driver Licensing Agency:
Georgia Department of Motor Vehicle Safety

P.O. Box 1456 | Atlanta, GA 30371
Tel: (678) 413-8400 | Web site: www.dds.ga.gov

Standard Length of license validation—4 years. Renewal options and conditions are in person. Vision testing is required at time of renewal, however, no written or road test is required.

Age-based renewal procedures—None

Reporting Procedures

Physician/medical reporting	Physicians should report patients with diagnosed conditions hazardous to driving and/or any handicap which would render the individual incapable of safely operating a motor vehicle.
Immunity	None
Legal protection	None
DMV follow-up	Medical evaluation and retest
Other reporting	Will accept information from anyone with knowledge that the driver may be medically or mentally unfit to drive.
Anonymity	None

Role of the Medical Advisory Board—The Medical Advisory Board advises agency personnel on individual medical reports and assists the agency in the decision-making process.
Georgia Department of Motor Vehicle Safety, Medical Unit
P.O. Box 80447 | Conyers, GA 30013

HAWAII

State Office on Aging

Hawaii Executive Office on Aging
No. 1 Capitol District | 250 South Hotel Street, Suite 406
Honolulu, HI 96813-2831 | Tel: (808) 586-0100 | Fax: (808) 586-0185

Driver Rehabilitation and Assessment Programs

Castle Performance and Rehabilitation Center
Harry and Jeanette Weinberg Medical Plaza and Wellness Center
642 Ulukahiki Street | Suite 100 | Kailua, HI 96734 | Tel: (808) 263-5303
Castle Professional Center | 46-001 Kamehameha Highway, Suite 103
Kāneʻohe, HI 96744 | Tel: (808) 247-1175

Rehabilitation Hospital of the Pacific
226 North Kuakini Street | Honolulu, HI 96817
Tel: (808) 531-3511 | Fax: (808) 544-3310

Straub Hospital Geriatric Medicine Department
888 South King Street | Honolulu, HI 96813 | Tel: (808) 522-4344

Veterans Affairs
459 Patterson Road | Honolulu, HI | Tel: (808) 433-0660

University of Hawaii Department of Geriatric Medicine - Kuakini
Medical Center
Hale Pulama Mau Building | 347 N Kuakini St. | Honolulu, HI 96817
Tel: (808) 523-8461

Hawaii Driving Regulations

Driver Licensing Agency
Honolulu Division of Motor Vehicles & Licensing, Driver License Branch
1199 Dillingham Boulevard, Bay A-101 | Honolulu, HI 96817
Tel: (808) 532-7730 | Web site: www.co.honolulu.h.us/csd

Standard Length of license validation—6 years. Renewal options and
conditions are in person or by mail. Vision testing is required at time of
renewal, however, no written test. A road test is required only if necessary.

Age-based renewal procedures—Drivers aged 15–17 renew every 4 years;
drivers aged 18–71 renew every 6 years. After age 72, drivers must renew
every 2 years.

Reporting Procedures
Physician/medical reporting	Permitted but not required
Immunity	None

Legal protection	None
DMV follow-up	Driver notified in writing of referral.
Other reporting	Will accept information from courts, police, other DMVs, and family members.
Anonymity	N/A

Role of the Medical Advisory Board—The MAB advises the DMV on medical issues regarding individual drivers. Actions are based on the reommendation of the majority.

Department of Transportation: (808) 692-7656

County of issue at

Honolulu: (808) 532-7730 | Hawaii: (808) 961-2222

Kauai: (808) 241-6550 | Maui: (808) 270-7363

IDAHO

State Office on Aging

Idaho Commission on Aging
3380 Americana Terrace, No. 120 | P.O. Box 83720
Boise, ID 83720-0007 | Tel: (208) 334-3833 | Fax: (208) 334-3033

Driver Rehabilitation and Assessment Programs

Bonner General Hospital Rehabilitation Services
520 North 3rd Avenue | P. O. Box 1448
Sandpoint, ID 83864 | Tel: (208) 263-1441

Idaho Elks Rehabilitation Hospital
600 Robins Road | P.O. Box 1100 | Boise, ID 83701
Tel: (208) 489-4816 | Fax: (208) 489-4058

Magic Valley Regional Medical Center
218 North 250 West | Jerome, ID 83338 | Tel: (208) 324-4474

Minidoka Memorial Hospital
1224 Eighth Street | Rupert, ID 83550 | Tel: (208) 436-0481

St. Alphonsus Regional Medical Center Rehabilitation Services
1055 N. Curtis Rd. | Boise, ID 83706 | Tel: (208) 378-2121

Idaho Driving Regulations

Driver Licensing Agency
Idaho Transportation Department | Division of Motor Vehicles, Driver
Services
P.O. Box 7129 | Boise, ID 83707 | Tel: (208) 334-8716
Web site: www.2.state.id.us/itd/dmv

Standard Length of license validation—4 years or 8 years if under 63 years
old. Renewal options and conditions are mail-in every other cycle. Vision
testing is required, but no written test. A road test is required only if
requested by examiner, law enforcement agency, family member or DMV.
An annual road test may be required to coincide with vision or medical re-
testing requirements.

Age-based renewal procedures—After age 69, no renewal by mail.

Reporting Procedures

Physician/medical reporting	Yes (not specified)
Immunity	None
Legal protection	A physician may not be sued for submitting required medical informa-tion to the department. Reports received by the Driver's License Advisory Board for the purpose of assisting the department in determin-ing whether a person is qualified to be licensed may not be used as evidence in any civil or criminal trial.
DMV *follow-up*	License suspended upon referral.
*Other reporting	Will accept information from family members, other DMVs, and law enforcement officers.
Anonymity	Not anonymous or confidential

Role of the Medical Advisory Board—The medical information submitted is
initially reviewed by employees within the Driver Support Division who

work specifically with medical cases. If there is a question whether to issue a license, the information is reviewed by the Driver's License Advisory Board, which is composed of a small group of representatives and the sheriff.
Tel: (208) 334-8736

ILLINOIS

State Office on Aging

Illinois Department on Aging
421 East Capitol Avenue | Springfield, IL 62701
Tel: (217) 785-2870 | Fax: (217) 785-4477

Driver Rehabilitation and Assessment Programs

C.O.R.E. Therapy Group
11243 W La Porte Rd. | Mokena, IL 60448 | Tel: (630) 922-9099
Web site: www.optimalmobilitysolutions.com

CRS Rehabilitation Specialists
9200 Claumet Ave, Suite N100 | Munster, IN 46321 | Tel: (219) 513-0500
8950 Gross Point Road, Suite D | Skokie, IL 60077 | Tel: (847) 967-5100
2245 Enterprise Drive, Suite 4514 | Westchester, IL 60154
Tel: (708) 531-0099

Buehler Center on Aging at Northwestern University's
Feinberg School of Medicine | 750 North Lake Shore Drive, Suite 601
Chicago, IL 60611 | Tel: (312) 503-3087 | Fax: (312) 503-5868

Department of Rehabilitation Services
1279 North Milwaukee Ave. 4th Floor | Chicago, IL 60622 |
Tel: (312) 292-4400

Illinois College of Optometry Low Vision Clinic
3241 South Michigan | Chicago, IL 60616 | Tel: (312) 949-7295

Institute of Physical Medicine and Rehabilitation-Occupational
Therapy
6501 North Sheridan Road | Peoria, IL 61614
Tel: (309) 692-8110 | Fax: (309) 692-8673

Hines Veteran Affairs Hospital
5th Ave/Roosevelt Rd. 117C - Driver Rehabilitation
Hines, IL 60141-5000 | Tel: (708) 202-8387 x24382

Loyola University Health System Balance Disorder Center
Oakbrook Terrace Medical Center | One South Summit Avenue
Oakbrook Terrace, IL 60181 | Tel: (708) 216-7985

Lutheran General Hospital - Occupational Therapy
1775 Dempster Street | Park Ridge, IL 60068
Tel: (708) 696-7061 | Fax: (708) 696-5597

Marianjoy Rehabilitation Hospital Driver Rehabilitation Program
26 W 171 Roosevelt Road | Wheaton, IL 60189
Tel: (630) 462-4076 | Fax: (630) 268-1595
Web site: www.marianjoy.org

Optimal Mobility Solutions
13416 South Sunflower Court | Plainfield, IL 60544
Tel: (630) 922-1600 | Fax: (630) 922-9099

Paulson Center for Rehabilitation
619 Plainfield Rd. | Willowbrook, IL 60521 | Tel: (630) 856-8200

Rehabilitation Institute of Chicago at Alexian Brothers Medical Center
Occupational Therapy | 935 Beisner Road | Elk Grove Village, IL 60007
Tel: (847) 437-5500 | Fax: (847) 228-6739

Rehabilitation Institute of Chicago Driver Rehabilitation Program
345 E Superior Street, Room 1500 | Chicago, IL 60611
Tel: (312) 238-6277 | Fax: (312) 238-6040

Rush University Medical Center - Johnston R. Bowman Health Center
710 S. Paulina Street, Suite 433 | Chicago, IL 60612 | Tel: (312) 942-7000

Schawb Rehabilitation Hospital
1401 South California Blvd. | Chicago, IL 60608 | Tel: (773) 522-5881

The University of Chicago Center for Comprehensive
Care and Research on Memory Disorders

Windermere Senior Health Center
Cornell and 56th Street | Chicago, IL 60637 | Tel: (773) 834-4340

Top Driver
1141 S. Arlington Heights Rd., Suite D | Arlington Heights, IL 60005
Tel: (847) 439-7132 x223 | Fax: (847) 439-7597
Web site: www.drive-now.com

Trinity Outpatient Rehabilitation Services
465 42nd Avenue, Suite 145 | East Moline, IL 61244
Tel: (309) 779-3490 | Fax: (309) 779-5615

Illinois Driving Regulations

Driver Licensing Agency
Illinois Office of the Secretary of State
Driver Services Department - Downstate
2701 S Dirksen Parkway | Springfield, IL 62723 | Tel: (217) 785 0963
Driver Services Department – Metro
17 N State Street, Suite 1100 | Chicago, IL 60602
Web site: www.sos.state.il.us/departments/drivers/drivers.html

Standard Length of license validation—4 years. Renewal options and
conditions are mail-in every other cycle for drivers with clean records and
no medical report. Vision testing is required at in-person renewal.. A
written test is required every 8 years unless driver has a clean driving
record. A road test is required only for applicants age 75+.

Age-based renewal procedures—Drivers age 75+: no renewal by mail; vision
test and on-road driving test required at each renewal. Drivers age 81–86:
renewal every 2 years. Drivers age 87+: renewal every year.

Reporting Procedures
   Physician/medical reporting   Physicians are encouraged to inform
patients of their responsibility to notify
the Secretary of State of any medical
conditions that may cause a loss of
consciousness or affect safe operation
of a motor vehicle within 10 days of
becoming aware of the condition.

Immunity	Yes
Legal protection	N/A (Illinois is not a mandatory reporting state)
DMV follow-up	The driver is notified in writing of the referral and required to submit a medical report. Determination of further action is based on various scenarios.
*Other reporting	Will accept information from courts, other DMVs, law enforcement agencies, members of the Illinois medical advisory board, National Driver Register (NDR), Problem Driver Pointer System, Secretary of State, management employees, Federal Motor Carrier Safety Administration, and driver rehabilitation specialists.
Anonymity	Available

Role of the Medical Advisory Board—The MAB reviews each medical report and determines the status of the licensee's driving privileges. The decision of the MAB is implemented by the Secretary of State. Supervisor, Medical Review Unit | Office of the Secretary of State Driver Services Department | 2701 South Dirksen Parkway Springfield, IL 62723 | Tel: (217) 785-3002

INDIANA

State Office on Aging

Indiana Bureau of Aging and In-Home Services
Division of Disability, Aging and Rehabilitative Services
Family and Services Administration | 402 W Washington Street
P.O. Box 7083 | Indianapolis, IN 46207-7083
Tel: (317) 232-7123 | Fax: (317) 232-7867

Driver Rehabilitation and Assessment Programs

Adaptive Mobility, Inc.
7050 North Guion Way | Indianapolis, IN 46268 | Tel: (317) 347-6400

Assistive Driving Services
681 W 1000 S. | Clayton, IN 46118
Tel: (317) 539-7012 | Fax: (317) 539-7013

Columbus Regional Hospital
1732 Timbercrest Dr. | Columbus, IN 47203
Tel: (800) 841-4938 x5902 | Fax: (812) 376-5941

Crossroads Rehabilitation Center
4740 Kingsway Drive | Indianapolis, IN 46205
Tel: (317) 466-1000 x2499 | Fax: (317) 466-2000
Web site: www.eastersealscrossroads.org

CRS Rehabilitation Specialists
9200 Calumet Avenue, Suite N100 | Munsyer, IN 46321
Tel: (219) 513-0500

Driver Rehabilitation Services
1718 Fisher Avenue | Warsaw, IN 46580
Toll Free: (800) 738-9967 | Fax: (219) 268-1112

Easter Seals Crossroads
4740 Kingsway Drive | Indianapolis, IN 46205
Tel: (317) 466-1000 x2536 | Fax: (317) 466-2000

Easter Seals Southwestern Indiana - The Rehabilitation Center
3701 Bellemeade Avenue | Evansville, IN 47714
Tel: (812) 479-1411 | Web site: www.eastersealsswindiana.com

Excel Driving Instruction
2403 North Campbell Street | Valparaiso, IN 46385 | Tel: (219) 548-2788

Hartford Center of Excellence in Geriatric Medicine
Indiana University School of Medicine
1001 West 10th Street, OPW M200 | Indianapolis, IN 46202
Tel: (317) 630-2219 | Fax: (317) 630-7066

Indiana State University Center for Driver Education
Department of Health Safety and Environmental Health Sciences
Arena B-76 | Terre Haute, IN 47809
Tel: (812) 237-3074 | Toll Free: (800) 654-6975 | Fax: (812) 237-4338

Indiana University Hospital Rehabilitation Services
550 University Blvd., Rm. 0102 | Indianapolis, IN 46202
Tel: (317) 962-9830 | Fax: (317) 962-9834

Indiana University School of Optometry
800 E Atwater Ave. | Bloomington, IN 47405-3680
Tel: (812) 855-4447 | Fax: (812) 855-8664

Margaret Mary Community Hospital
321 Mitchell Ave., Box 226 | Batesville, IN 47006
Tel: (812) 934-6512 | Fax: (812) 934-6122

Memorial Hospital - Memorial Outpatient Therapy Services
111 W Jefferson, Suite 100 | South Bend, IN 46601
Tel: (574) 647-2634 | Fax: (574) 239-6460

Regional Rehab Driving, Inc.
P.O. Box 298 | Schererville, IN 46375
Tel: (219) 718-2366 | Fax: (219) 322-6530

Rehabilitation Hospital of Indiana Neurological Rehabilitation Center
9531 Valaparaiso | Indianapolis, IN 46268
Tel: (317) 878-8940 | Fax: (317) 872-0914

Richard L. Roudebush Veteran Affairs Medical Center
1481 W Tenth Street | Indianapolis, IN 46202 | Tel: (317) 554-0000

The Low Vision Centers of Indiana
Indianapolis Office Tel: (317) 844-0919
Fort Wayne Office Tel: (260) 432-0575
Hartford City Tel: (765) 348-2020

The Rehabilitation Center
3701 Bellemeade Avenue | Evansville, IN 47714-0161
Tel: (812) 479-1411

Therapeutic Mobility Services
7603 Kilbourn Drive | Ft. Wayne, IN 46809
Tel: (260) 747-4758 | Fax: (260) 747-4801

Indiana Driving Regulations

Driver Licensing Agency
Indiana Bureau of Motor Vehicles, Driver Services
100 N Senate Avenue, Rm. N 405 | Indianapolis, IN 46204
Web site: www.in.gov/bmv

Standard Length of license validation—4 to 6 years if under 75.3 years for
ages 75 to 85 and over 85, 2 years. Renewal options in person with a vision
test required at time of renewal (acuity and peripheral fields). A road test is
required only for those with 14+ points or 3 convictions in 12-month
period.

Age-based renewal procedures—At age 75, renewal cycle is reduced to
3 years.

Reporting Procedures

Physician/medical reporting	None. However, there is a statute requiring that physicians and others who diagnose, treat, or provide care for handicapped persons report the handicapping condition to the state Board of Health within 60 days.
Immunity	None
Legal protection	N/A
DMV follow-up	Driver notified in writing of referral.
*Other reporting	Will accept information from courts, police, other DMVs, family members, and other sources.
Anonymity	N/A

Role of the Medical Advisory Board—The MAB advises the Bureau of
Motor Vehicles on medical issues regarding individual drivers. Actions are
based on the recommendation of the majority and/or specialist.

IOWA

State Office on Aging

Iowa Department of Elder Affairs
Clemens Building, 3rd Floor | 200 Tenth Street
Des Moines, IA 50309-3609 | Tel: (515) 242-3333 | Fax: (515) 242-3300

Driver Rehabilitation and Assessment Programs

Department of Veterans Affairs Rehabilitation Medicine Service
1515 West Pleasant, Department 117A | Knoxville, IA 50138
Tel: (515) 842-3101 | Fax: (515) 828-5120

Genesis Medical Center
1227 E Rusholme St. | Davenport, IA 52803
Tel: (563) 421-1405 | Fax: (563) 421-1410
Web site: www.genesishealth.com

Iowa Joint Center at Jennie Edmundson Hospital
933 E Pierce St. | Council Bluffs, IA 51503 | Tel: (712) 396-4495

Iowa Program for Assistive Technology (IPAT)
Center for Disabilities and Development | 100 Hawkins Drive, Room S295
Iowa City, IA 52242-1011 | Tel: (319) 356-0550 | Toll Free: (800) 331-3027

Mercy Medical Center - North Iowa
186 North Crescent Drive | Mason City, IA 50401 | Tel: (641) 422-7724

St. Luke's Hospital - Occupational Therapy
1026 A Avenue NE | P.O. Box 3026 | Cedar Rapids, IA 52406
Tel: (319) 369-7278 | Fax: (319) 369-8186

The Finley Hospital Outpatient Rehab
444 N Grandview Ave. | Dubuque, IA 52001 | Tel: (563) 589-2497
3365 Hillcrest Road | Dubuque, IA 52002 | Tel: (563) 557-9955

Trinity Regional Medical Center Rehabilitation Services
802 Kenyon Road | Fort Doge, IA 50501 | Tel: (515) 573-3101

University of Iowa Hospitals & Clinics
Memory Disorders Clinic - Department of Neurology

200 Hawkins Drive, 2155 RCP | Iowa City, IA 52242
Tel: (319) 356-0872 | Fax: (319) 356-4505
Benton Neuropsychology Laboratory of Neurology
Tel: (319) 356-2671 or (877) 384-8999

Younker Rehabilitation Center - Occupational Therapy
1200 Pleasant St. | Des Moines, IA 50309
Tel: (515) 241-8139 | Fax: (515) 241-5137

Iowa Driving Regulations

Driver Licensing Agency
Iowa Motor Vehicle Division | Park Fair Mall, 100 Euclid Avenue
P.O. Box 9201 | Des Moines, IA 50306-9204
Tel: (515) 244-8725 or (800) 532-1121 | Web site: www.dot.state.ia.us/mvd

Standard Length of license validation—5 years, in person, extensions
available if out of state for 6 months. Vision testing is required at time of
renewal, however, no written test required. A road test is required if
physical or mental conditions are present.

Age-based renewal procedures—Persons under the age of 18 or aged 70 and
older are issued 2-year licenses.

Reporting Procedures

Physician/medical reporting	A physician may report to the motor vehicle division "the identity of a person who has been diagnosed as having a physical or mental condition which would render the person physically or mentally incompetent to operate a motor vehicle in a safe manner."
Immunity	Available
Legal protection	Under 321 186, "a physician or optometrist making a report shall be immune from any liability, civil or criminal, which might otherwise be incurred or imposed as a result of the report."
DMV follow-up	Driver notified in writing of referral. License suspended upon referral.

| *Other reporting | Will accept information from courts, other DMVs, police, and family members. |
| *Anonymity | Not anonymous or confidential |

Role of the Medical Advisory Board—The MAB reviews medical/vision reports as requested and makes recommendations regarding the individual's capability to drive safely.

Iowa Medical Society | 1001 Grand Avenue
West Des Moines, IA 50265-3502 | Tel: (515) 223-1401

KANSAS

State Office on Aging

Kansas Department on Aging
New England Building | 503 South Kansas Avenue
Topeka, KS 66603-3404
Tel: (785) 296-5222 | Fax: (785) 296-0256

Driver Rehabilitation and Assessment Programs

Human Motion Institute Rehabilitation Services at Overland Park
Regional
12200 W 106th Street, Suite 430 | Overland Park, KS 66215
Tel: (913) 541-5001 | Fax: (913) 541-5003

Kansas Rehabilitation Hospital
1504 SW 8th Street | Topeka, KS 66606
Tel: (785) 235-6600 | Fax: (785) 232-8509

Lawrence Rehabilitation Clinic
3511 Clinton Place | Lawrence, KS 66047 | Tel: (785) 331-3783

Meadowbrook Rehabilitation Hospital
427 West Main | Gardner, KS 66030-1183
Tel: (913) 856-8747 | Fax: (913) 856-8339

Shawnee Mission Medical Center - TherapyPlus
9120 W 75th Street | Shawnee Mission, KS 66204 | Tel: (913) 676-2444

The University of Kansas Medical Center
3901 Rainbow Boulevard | Kansas City, KS 66160 | Tel: (913) 588-5000

Via Christi Rehabilitation Center - Our Lady of Lourdes
1151 N Rock Rd. | Wichita, KS 67206 | Tel: (316) 634-3400

Wesley Rehabilitation Hospital
8338 West 13th St. N | Wichita, KS 67212 | Tel: (316) 729-9999

Kansas Driving Regulations

Driver Licensing Agency
Kansas Division of Motor Vehicles | Docking State Office Building
P.O. Box 2188 | Topeka, KS 66601-2128
Tel: (785) 296-3963 | Fax: (785) 296-0691
Web site: www.accesskansas.org/living/cars-transportation.html

Standard Length of license validation—6 years, renewal in person. A vision test is required at time of renewal, along with a written test. A road test is required by the examiner challenge, for visual acuity of 20/60 or worse, or at medical doctor's request.

Age-based renewal procedures—At age 65, renewal cycle is reduced to 4 years.

Reporting Procedures

Physician/medical reporting	Statutes specify that physicians are not required to volunteer information to the division or to the medical advisory board concerning the mental or physical condition of any patient.
Legal protection	Patients must sign a form permitting the MD or OD to release information to the DMV. Persons so reporting in good faith are statutorily immunized from civil actions for damages caused by such reporting.
DMV *follow-up*	Driver is notified in writing of referral.
*Other reporting	Will accept information from courts, other DMVs, police, family members, and concerned citizens.

Anonymity	Letters of concern must be signed.
	Applicants may request a copy of the letter.

Role of the Medical Advisory Board—The MAB assists the Director of Vehicles and Driver Review in interpreting conflicting information and formulating action based on the recommendation of specialists. It also helps determine the driving eligibility of complicated or borderline cases.
Kansas Driver Review | Medical Advisory Board
915 SW Harrison, Room 162 | Topeka, KS 66626

KENTUCKY

State Office on Aging

Kentucky Office of Aging Services
Cabinet for Health Services | 275 East Main Street, 5C-D
Frankfort, KY 40621
Tel: (502) 564-6930 | Fax: (502) 564-4595

Driver Rehabilitation and Assessment Programs

Baptist Rehabilitation Center
115 Kiana Court | Paducah, KY | Tel: (270) 534-1200

Bryant Driving School
Louisville, KY | Tel: (502) 288-7211 | Toll Free: (800) 76-DRIVE

Cardinal Hill Rehabilitation Hospital
2050 Versailles Rd. | Lexington, KY 40504 | Tel: (859) 367-7125

Department of Vocational Rehabilitation
2052 Glade Lane | Lexington, KY 40513
Tel: (859) 223-5826 | Fax: (859) 223-5826

Frazier Rehabilitation Institute - Newburg ORF
3430 Newburg Rd., Ste. 111A | Louisville, KY 40220
Tel: (502) 451-6886 | Fax: (502) 458-2158

Gateway Rehabilitation Hospital at Florence
5940 Merchants Street | Florence, KY 41042 | Tel: (859) 426-2400

HEALTHSOUTH Northern Kentucky Rehabilitation Hospital
201 Medical Village Drive | Edgewood, KY 41017 | Tel: (859)341-2044

Kentucky Office for the Blind
P. O. Box 210 | Prospect, KY 40059 | Tel: (502) 396-5721

Rehabilitation Hospital of Central Kentucky
134 Heartland Drive | Elizabethtown, KY 42701 | Tel: (270) 769-3100

Samaritan Hospital - Occupational Therapy
310 South Limestone Street | Lexington, KY 40508 | Tel: (859) 226-7000

University of Kentucky Medical Center - Kentucky Clinic - J111
Physical Therapy / Occupational Therapy Department
Lexington, KY 40536 | Tel: (859) 881-3773 | Fax: (859) 246-2124

University of Kentucky Driving Program
800 Rose Street HP500A | Lexington, KY 40536 | Tel: (859) 608-4959

Veteran Affairs Healthcare Center, Grade Lane
Air National Guard Complex | 1101 Grade Lane
Louisville, KY | Tel: (502) 364-9635

Kentucky Driving Regulations

Driver Licensing Agency
Kentucky Division of Driver Licensing
501 High Street | Frankfort, KY 40602 | Tel: (502) 564-6800
Web site: www.kytc.state.ky.us/drlic

Standard Length of license validation—4 years, in-person. There are no
vision, written, or road tests.

Age-based renewal procedures—None

Reporting Procedures
    Physician/medical reporting   Yes (not specified)
    Immunity   Yes
    Legal protection   None

DMV follow-up	Driver is notified in writing of referral to medical advisory board.
*Other reporting	Will accept information from courts, other DMVs, family members, and police.
Anonymity	None

Role of the Medical Advisory Board—The medical advisory board identifies drivers with physical or mental impairments that impede their ability to safely operate a motor vehicle.
Tel: (502) 564-6800 x2552 | Fax: (502) 564-6145

LOUISIANA

State Office on Aging

Governor's Office of Elderly Affairs
P.O. Box 80374 | 412 N 4th Street | Baton Rouge, LA 70802
Tel: (225) 342-7100 | Fax: (225) 342-7133

Driver Rehabilitation and Assessment Programs

Association of Driver Educators for the Disabled
711 S Vienna Street | Ruston, LA 71270
Tel: (318) 257-5055 | Toll Free: (800) 290-2344 | Fax: (318) 255-4175
Web site: http://www.aded.net

Driving Rehab Solutions, LLC
1035 Masterson Drive | Baton Rouge, LA 70810
Tel: (225) 751-3379 | Fax: (225) 751-3363
Web site: www.drivingrehabsolutions.com

Louisiana Center for the Blind
101 South Trenton | Ruston, LA 71270
Tel: (318) 251-2891 | Toll Free: (800) 234-4166

Louisiana Rehabilitation Services
8225 Florida Boulevard | Baton Rouge, LA 70806-4834
Tel: (504) 925-4131

Luling Rehabilitation Hospital
1125 Paul Maillard | Luling, LA 70070 | Tel: (985) 331-2281

North Oaks Rehabilitation Hospital
1900 S Morrison Blvd. | Hammond, LA 70403 | Tel: (985) 345-2700

Our Lady of Lourdes Hospital - Outpatient Rehabilitation Program
611 St. Landry Street | Lafayette, LA 70506
Tel: (337) 289-2859 | Fax: (337) 289-2883

Sterlington Rehabilitation Hospital
111 LA Highway 2 | Sterlington, LA 71280 | Tel: (318) 665-9950

United Medical Rehabilitation Hospital
5650 Read Boulevard | New Orleans, LA 70127
Tel: (504)242-4246 | Fax: (504)240-6618

Louisiana Driving Regulations

Driver Licensing Agency
Louisiana Office of Motor Vehicles
P.O. Box 64886 | Baton Rouge, LA 70896
Tel: (877) 368-5463 | Web site: www.expresslane.org

Standard Length of license validation—4 years. Renewal options and conditions are in person or by mail every other cycle. Renewal can also be done by Internet and interactive voice response, unless license has been expired 6 months or more. A vision test is required at time of renewal. A written test is required if license has been expired 1 year or more and a road test is required if license has been expired 2 years or more.

Age-based renewal procedures—No renewal by mail for drivers over the age of 70.

Reporting Procedures
    Physician/medical reporting   If the applicant's ability to drive safely is questionable, it is desired, but not required to report patients. However, if a medical report is filed, it must address the medical concern for which it was

	required; contain the physician's signature, address, and phone number; and be dated within 60 days from the date received by the Department.
Immunity	A physician who provides such information has statutory immunity from civil or criminal liability for damages arising out of an accident.
Legal protection	Louisiana has statutory protection for good faith reporting of unsafe drivers.
DMV follow-up	Driver is notified in writing of referral.
*Other reporting	Will accept information from DMV employees or agents in the performance of duties, law enforcement officers, health care providers, or family members.
Anonymity	Not anonymous or confidential. However, an order from a court of competent jurisdiction is required before the identity of the reporter can be released.

Role of the Medical Advisory Board—Medical reports requiring further attention are forwarded to the Data Prep Unit marked Attention: Conviction/Medical Unit. The conviction/medical unit evaluates these reports and may request an evaluation by the MAB. The MAB then recommends actions.

MAINE

State Office on Aging

Maine Bureau of Elder and Adult Services - Department of Human Services
442 Civic Center Drive | 11 State House Station | Augusta, ME 04333-0011
Tel: (207) 287-9200 | Fax: (207) 287-9229

Driver Rehabilitation and Assessment Programs

Alpha 1 Driver Evaluation Program
127 Maine Street | South Portland, ME 04106
Tel: (207) 767-2189 | Fax: (207) 799-8346

Eastern Maine Medical Center - Maine Rehabilitation Center
489 State St. | Bangor, ME 04401 | Tel: (207) 973-8815

Mercy Health Center Physical Rehabilitation
616 Forest Avenue | Portland, ME | Tel: (207) 771-1730

New England Rehabilitation Hospital of Portland
335 Brighton Avenue | Portland, ME 04102-2374 | Tel: (207) 662-8377

Southern Maine Medical Center - The Memory Clinic
72 Main Street | Kennebunk, ME 04043 Tel: (207) 467-6987

St. Mary's Regional Medical Center - Club 50
Campus Avenue | P.O. Box 291 | Lewiston, ME 04243-0291
Tel: (207) 777-8823

University of New England College of Osteopathic Medicine
Maine Geriatric Education Center | 11 Hills Beach Road
Biddeford, ME 04005-9599

Maine Driving Regulations

Driver Licensing Agency
Maine Bureau of Motor Vehicles | 101 Hospital Street
Augusta, ME 04333-0029
Tel: (207) 624-9000 | Web site: www.state.me.us/sos/bmv

Standard Length of license validation—6 years. Vision tested at age 40, 52, 65, and every 4 years thereafter. There is no written or road test at time of renewal.

Age-based renewal procedures—At age 65, the license renewal cycle is reduced to every 4 years.

Reporting Procedures
Physician/medical reporting	Yes (not specified)
Immunity	N/A
Legal protection	A physician acting in good faith is immune from any damages as a result of the filing of a certificate of examination.

DMV *follow-up*	The DMV will require a medical evaluation form to be completed by a physician at periodic intervals.
*Other reporting	Will accept information from courts, other DMVs, police, family members, and other sources.
Anonymity	Not anonymous or confidential. The identity of the reporter may be revealed at an administrative hearing if requested.

Role of the Medical Advisory Board—The Medical Advisory Board reviews the medical information submitted whenever an individual contests an action of the Division of Driver Licenses. Reports received or made by the Board are confidential and may not be disclosed unless the individual gives written permission. Tel: (207) 624-9101

MARYLAND

State Office on Aging

Maryland Department of Aging
301 West Preston Street, Suite 1007
Baltimore, MD 21201
Tel: (410) 767-1100 | Fax: (410) 333-7943

Driver Rehabilitation and Assessment Programs

Adventist Rehabilitation Hospital
9909 Medical Center Drive | Rockville, MD 20850
Tel: (240) 864-6000 | Fax: (240) 864-6144
831 E University Boulevard | Silver Spring, MD 20903
Tel: (301) 445-3191 | Fax: (301) 445-3198
7600 Carroll Ave – Unit 5200 | Takoma Park, MD 20912
Tel: (301) 891-5560 | Fax: (301) 891-5111

Anne Arundel Community College
GBTC, 101 N Crain Highway | Glen Burnie, MD 21061-3060
Tel: (410) 777-2939 | Fax: (410) 777-2979

American Occupational Therapy Association (AOTA)
4720 Montgomery Lane | Bethesda, MD 20824
Tel: (952) 942-8859 | Fax: (952) 942-7673

Blind Industries and Services of Maryland
2901 Strickland Street | Baltimore, MD 21223 | Tel: (410) 233-4567

Department of Veterans Affairs BRECC - VAMC
13505 Winding Trail Court | Silver Spring, MD 20906 |
Tel: (301) 603-0255

Driving Rehabilitation of Frederick, Inc.
85 Thomas Johnson Court, Suite B | Frederick, MD 21702 |
Tel: (301) 682-9110

Good Samaritans Hospital Rehabilitation Services
5601 Loch Raven Blvd. | Baltimore, MD 21239 | Tel: (410) 532-4701

HEALTHSOUTH Chesapeake Rehabilitation Hospital
220 Tilghman Road | Salisbury, MD 21804 | Tel: (410) 546-4600

Sinai Rehabilitation Center, Sinai Hospital
2401 W. Belvedere Ave. | Baltimore, MD 21215-5271
Tel: (410) 601-9843 | Fax: (410) 601-9080
Web site: www.lifebridgehealth.org

Technology Assistance Program
2301 Argonne Drive, Rm T-17 | Baltimore, MD 21218
Tel: (410) 554-9230 | Toll Free: (800) 832-4827

University of Maryland Medical Center - Division of Gerontology
22 South Greene Street | Baltimore, MD 21201

Maryland Driving Regulations

Driver Licensing Agency
Maryland Motor Vehicle Administration | 6601 Ritchie Highway, NE
Glen Burnie, MD 21062 | Tel: (301) 729-4500 or (800) 950-1682
Web site: www.mva.state.md.us

Standard Length of license validation—5 years, renewal in person. Vision testing is required at time of renewal (visual acuity and visual fields), however, no written or road test is required.

Age-based renewal procedures—Medical report required for new drivers age 70 and older.

Reporting Procedures

Physician/medical reporting	Maryland law provides for the discretionary reporting to the Motor Vehicle Administration of persons who have "disorders characterized by lapses of consciousness."
Immunity	N/A
Legal protection	A civil or criminal action may not be brought against any person who makes a report to the Medical Advisory Board and who does not violate any confidential or privileged relationship conferred by law.
DMV follow-up	Driver is notified in writing of referral. License is suspended and further examination is required.
*Other reporting	Will accept information from courts, other DMVs, police, family members, and other sources.
Anonymity	Confidentiality available if requested by reporter.

Role of the Medical Advisory Board—The MAB advises the Motor Vehicle Administration on medical issues regarding individual drivers. Actions are based on the recommendation of the majority and/or specialist. Tel: (410) 768-7513

MASSACHUSETTS

State Office on Aging

Massachusetts Executive Office of Elder Affairs
One Ashburton Place | Boston, MA 02108
Tel: (617) 222-7451 | Fax: (617) 727-6944

Driver Rehabilitation and Assessment Programs

Adaptive Driving Program, Inc.
250 Milton Street, #LL002 | Dedham, MA 02026-2904
Tel: (781) 329-6656 | Fax: (781) 329-6390

Beth Israel Deaconess Medical Center
DriveWise: A driving fitness evaluation program
330 Brookline Ave. | Boston, MA 02215 | Tel: (617) 667-4074

Driving Solutions
8 Marshall Street | North Reading, MA 01864 | Tel: (978) 664-2686

Fairlawn Rehabilitation Hospital - Driving Evaluations Clinic
189 May Street | Worcester, MA 01602 | Tel: (508) 791-6351

Hebrew Rehabilitation Center
1200 Centre Street | Boston, MA 02131 | Tel: (617) 363-8000

Jewish Memorial Hospital and Rehabilitation Center
59 Townsend Street | Boston, MA 02119
Tel: (617) 989-8315 | Fax: (617) 989-8207

Massachusetts Eye and Ear Infirmary - Vision Rehabilitation Center
243 Charles Street | Boston, MA 02114 | Tel: (617) 573-4177

New England Sinai Hospital and Rehabilitation Center
150 York Street | Stoughton, MA 02072 | Tel: (781) 344-0600

Rehabilitation Hospital of the Cape and Islands
RoadSMART Driver Rehabilitation Program
RHCI-SANDWICH Outpatient Rehabilitation Center
311 Service Road | East Sandwich, MA 02537 | Tel: (508) 833–4110

RHCI-BOURNE Outpatient Rehabilitation Center
One Technology Park Drive, Suite A | Upper Cape Medical and
Business Park | Bourne, MA 02532
Tel: (508) 743–0465

Shaughnessy-Kaplan Rehabilitation Hospital
Driver Evaluation and Retraining Program
Dove Avenue | Salem, MA 01970 | Tel: (978) 825-8513

Spaulding Rehabilitation Hospital - Occupational Therapy
125 Nashua Street | Boston, MA 02114
Tel: (617) 720-6624 | Fax: (617) 720-6630

Veteran Affairs Boston Healthcare System
1400 VFW Parkway PMRS 117 | West Roxbury, MA 02370
Tel: (616) 323-7700 | Fax: (616) 363-5680

Weldon Rehabilitation Hospital Driver Advisement Program
3 Brentwood Drive | Wilbraham, MA 01095
Tel: (413) 596-6216

Whittier Rehabilitation Hospital
76 Summer Street | Haverhill, MA 01830
Tel: (978) 372-8000 | Fax: (978) 374-4423
150 Flanders Road | P.O. Box 1250 | Westborough, MA 01581
Tel: (508) 870-2222 | Fax: (508) 871-2048

Massachusetts Driving Regulations

Driver Licensing Agency
Massachusetts Registry of Motor Vehicles | P.O. Box 199100
Boston, MA 02119-9100 | Tel: (617) 351-4500
Web site: www.state.ma.us/rmv

Standard Length of license validation—5 years, renewal options are in
person or via Internet. A vision test is required at renewal. No written or
road test is required, however, DMV reviews on a case-by-case basis and
will administer a written or road test if indicated.

Age-based renewal procedures—None

Reporting Procedures

Physician/medical reporting	Massachusetts is a self-reporting state. It is the responsibility of the driver to report to the Registry of Motor Vehicles any medical condition that may impair driving ability. However, physicians are encouraged to report unfit drivers to the Registry of Motor Vehicles.
Immunity	N/A
Legal protection	The law does not provide any protection from liability, nor does it promise confidentiality due to the "Public Records" law which states simply that a driver is entitled to any information upon receipt of written approval.
DMV follow-up	If the report comes from the general public or a family member, it must be in writing and signed. If the report is accepted, the driver is contacted by mail and asked to obtain medical clearance to certify that he/she is safe to drive. If the DMV does not receive a response within 30 days, a second request is mailed. If there is still no response, then the license is revoked. If the report is from a law enforcement officer or physician, it is considered an "immediate threat." The driver is contacted by mail and requested to voluntarily surrender his/her license or submit medical clearance within 10 days. If there is no response, then the license is revoked.
*Other reporting	Will accept information from courts, other DMVs, police, family members, and other sources.
Anonymity	None

Role of the Medical Advisory Board—The MAB provides guidance to the Registry of Motor Vehicles when there are medical issues relating to an applicant's eligibility for a learner's permit or driver's license, or when an individual's privilege to operate a motor vehicle has been—or is in danger of being—restricted, suspended, or revoked.

Massachusetts Registry of Motor Vehicles | Medical Affairs Bureau
P.O. Box 199100 | Boston, MA 02119-9100 | Tel: (617) 351-9222
Web site: www.state.ma.us/rmv

MICHIGAN

State Office on Aging

Michigan Office of Services to the Aging
P.O. Box 30676
7109 West Saginaw, First Floor
Lansing, MI 48909-8176
Tel: (517) 373-8230 | Fax: (517) 373-4092

Driver Rehabilitation and Assessment Programs

Disability Resource Center of Southwest Michigan
Driver Rehabilitation & Driver Training | 517 E Crosstown Pkwy
Kalamazoo, MI 49001-2867 | Tel: (269) 345-1516 | Fax: (269) 345-0229
Web site: www.drccil.org

Drivers Rehabilitation Center of Michigan
28911 Seven Mile Road | Livonia, MI 48152
Tel: (734) 422-3000 | Fax: (734) 432-6007 | Web site: www.AA-Driving.com

Driver Rehabilitation Systems, Inc.
11643 S Saginaw, Suite 1A | Grand Blanc, MI 48439 | Tel: (810) 694-9830

Independent Living Services, Inc.
199 North Maine Street, Suite 101 | Plymouth, MI 48170
Tel: (734) 254-0125

Irish Hills Mobility
12745 North Crystal Lake Drive | Cement City, MI 49233
Tel: (517) 206-3837

Mary Free Bed Rehabilitation Hospital
235 Wealthy St. SE | Grand Rapids, MI 49503-5299
Tel: (616) 456-4856 | Fax: (616) 451-9513 | Web site: www.maryfreebed.com

Munson Medical Center - Occupational Therapy Department
1105 Sixth St. | Traverse City, MI 49684
Tel: (231) 935-7350 | Fax: (231) 935-7344

Rehabilitation Institute of Michigan Novi Center
42005 W 12 Mile | Novi, MI 48377
Tel: (248) 305-7575 | Fax: (248) 305-7556 | Web site: www.rimrehab.org

Saginaw Community Hospital - Driver Evaluation and Training Program
3340 Hospital Road | P.O. Box 6280 | Saginaw, MI 48608
Tel: (517) 790-7819 | Fax: (517) 790-7818

St. Joseph Murphy of Macomb - Occupational Therapy
15855 Nineteen Mile Road | Clinton TWP, MI 48038
Tel: (313) 263-2489 | Fax: (313) 263-2490

Southwest Rehabilitation Hospital
183 West Street | Battle Creek, MI 49017 | Tel: (269) 964-5808

Special Driving Services, Inc.
P.O. Box 241 | Okemos, MI 48805
Tel: (517) 321-7176 | Fax: (517) 349-7990

University of Michigan Drive - Ability Program
Medrehab 355 Briarwood Circle #4 | Ann Arbor, MI 48160
Tel: (734) 998-7911 or (734) 998-7914 | Fax: (734) 998-9429

Veterans Affairs Medical Center–Allen Park Occupational Therapy
Southfield and Outer Drive | Allen Park, MI 48101 | Tel: (313) 562-6000

William Beaumont Health Center Driver Rehab Program
4949 Coolidge Highway | Royal Oak, MI 48073
Tel: (248) 655-5800 | Fax: (248) 655-5801

Michigan Driving Regulations

Driver Licensing Agency
Michigan Department of State | 7707 Rickle Road | Lansing, MI 48918
Tel: (517) 322-1460 | Web site: www.michigan.gov/sos

Standard Length of license validation—4 years. For renewal options and conditions one can mail in every other cycle, if free of convictions. There is a vision and written test at time of renewal, and a road test if the license has been expired more than 4 years.

Age-based renewal procedures—No

Reporting Procedures

Physician/medical reporting	Physicians are encouraged to report unsafe drivers. They may do so by completing a "Request for Driver Evaluation" form (OC-88). This form can be downloaded from the Michigan Department of State Web site.
Immunity	None
Legal protection	None
DMV follow-up	The driver is notified in writing of the referral. The notification includes a notice of date, time, and location of driver reexamination as well as any medical statements to be completed by the driver's doctor.
*Other reporting	The Department accepts referrals for reexamination from family, police, public officials, and others who have knowledge of a driver's inability to drive safely or health concerns that may affect his/her driving ability.
Anonymity	Reporting is not anonymous. However, the Department will release the name of the reporter only if he/she is a public official (e.g., police, judge, state employee). The names of non-public official reporters will be released only under court order.

Role of the Medical Advisory Board—The MAB advises the Department of State on medical issues regarding individual drivers. Actions are based on the recommendation of specialists.

Driver Assessment Office | Tel: (517) 241-6840

MINNESOTA

State Office on Aging

Minnesota Board on Aging - Aging and Adult Services Division
P.O. Box 64976 V | St. Paul, MN 55164-0976
Tel: (651) 431-2500 | Toll Free: (800) 882-6262 | Fax: (651) 431-7453

Driver Rehabilitation and Assessment Programs

Bethesda Rehabilitation Hospital
2512 S 7th St., 4th Floor | Minneapolis, MN 55454 | Tel: (651) 326-1000
559 Capitol Blvd. | St. Paul, MN 55103 | Tel: (651) 232-2000

BLIND, Incorporated
100 East 22nd Street South | Minneapolis, MN 55404
Tel: (612) 872-0100

Courage Center
3915 Golden Valley Road | Golden Valley, MN 55422
Tel: (763) 520-0435 | Fax: (763) 520-0355
Web site: www.courage.org

Drive Safe
4807 Kings Crossing N | Brooklyn Park, MN 55443-3999
Tel: (651) 343-1335 | Fax: (763) 425-6444

Occupational Therapy Solutions, Inc.
1612 East Minnehaha Parkway | Minneapolis, MN 55407
Tel: (612) 722-5815

Sister Kenny Rehabilitation Institute Driving Simulator
800 E 28th St. | Minneapolis, MN 55407 | Tel: (612) 863-4466

SPOT Rehabilitation Driver Review Program
2835 W St. Germain #300 | P.O. Box 7729 | St. Cloud, MN 56301-7729
Tel: (320) 259-4151 | Toll Free: (888) 404-7768 | Fax: (320) 259-5707

The Center for Independent Living of Northeastern Minnesota
Mesabi Mall, Suite 25 | 1101 East 37th Street | Hibbing, MN 55746
Tel: (218) 262-6675 | Toll Free: (800) 390-3681 | Fax: (218) 262-6677

Minnesota Driving Regulations

Driver Licensing Agency
Minnesota Department of Public Safety | Driver and Vehicle Services
445 Minnesota Street | St. Paul, MN 55101 | Tel: (651) 296-6911
Web site: www.dps.state.mn.us/dvs

Standard Length of license validation—4 years. Renewal options and
conditions are in person where a vision test is required. A written test is
required only if license has been expired for more than 1 year and a road
test is required only if license has been expired for more than 5 years.

Age-based renewal procedures—None

Reporting Procedures

Physician/medical reporting	Physician reporting is encouraged. Physicians may contact the Medical Unit in writing; no specific form is required.
Immunity	Yes
Legal protection	Not addressed in driver licensing laws.
DMV follow-up	Driver is notified in writing of referral. License is suspended upon referral and further examination is conducted.
*Other reporting	Will accept information from courts, other DMVs, police, family members, or other sources.
Anonymity	Reporting cannot be done anonymously. However, the identity of the reporter will be held confidential unless the court subpoenas records.

Role of the Medical Advisory Board—The MAB advises the Department of Public Safety on medical issues regarding individual drivers. Actions are based on the recommendation of the majority.

Minnesota Department of Public Safety

Medical Unit 445 Minnesota Street, Suite 170 | St. Paul, MN 55101-5170

Tel: (651) 296-2021

MISSISSIPPI

State Office on Aging

Mississippi Council on Aging - Division of Aging and Adult Services
750 North State Street | Jackson, MS 39202
Tel: (601) 359-4925 | Fax: (601) 359-4370

Driver Rehabilitation and Assessment Programs

Baptist Health Systems - Outpatient Rehab Services
1190 North State Street | Jackson, MS 39202
Tel: (601) 968-1148 | Fax: (601) 968-1337

Gulf Coast Veterans Health Care System - Rehabilitation Medical Services
400 Veterans Blvd. | Biloxi, MS 39591 | Tel: (601) 388-5541

Methodist Outpatient Rehabilitation Center
One Layfair Drive, Suite 110 | Flowood, MS 39232
Tel: (601) 936-8889 | Fax: (601) 936-8865
Web site: www.methodistonline.org

North Mississippi Medical Center - Occupational Therapy
830 South Gloster Street | Tupelo, MS 38801
Tel: (601) 841-4058 | Fax: (601) 842-8693

Rush Foundation Hospital - Occupational Therapy
1314 19th Avenue | Meridian, MS 39301 | Tel: (601) 703-4240

T.K. Martin Center for Technology & Disability
P. O. Box 9736 | Mississippi State, MS 39762
Tel: (662) 325-1028 | Fax: (662) 325-0896
Web site: www.tkmartin.msstate.edu
Southwest Center for Rehabilitation
Tel: (601) 249-4758

Mississippi Driving Regulations

Driver Licensing Agency
Mississippi Department of Public Safety | Driver Services
1900 E Woodrow Wilson | Jackson, MS 39216
Web site: www.dps.state.ms.us

Standard Length of license validation—4 years. Renewal options and conditions are in person; renewal via Internet permitted every other cycle. Vision test is required at time of renewal.

Age-based renewal procedures—None
Reporting Procedures

Physician/medical reporting	Permitted but not required
Immunity	No
Legal protection	N/A
DMV follow-up	N/A
*Other reporting	Will accept information from courts, other DMVs, police, and family members.
Anonymity	N/A

Role of the Medical Advisory Board—Mississippi does not retain a medical advisory board.

MISSOURI

State Office on Aging

Missouri Division of Senior & Disability Services
Department of Health & Senior Services
P.O. Box 570 | Jefferson City, MO 65102-0570
Tel: (573) 526-3626 | Fax: (573) 751-8687

Driver Rehabilitation and Assessment Programs

Adaptive Mobility, Inc.
116 Algana Court | St. Peters, MO 63376 | Tel: (636) 926-2225

Barnes Jewish Hospital Department of Geriatrics
One Barnes-Jewish Hospital Plaza | St. Louis, MO 63110
Tel: (314) 867-3627 | Toll Free. (866) 867-3627

Driving Rehabilitation Services
660 North New Ballas | St. Louis, MO 63141
Tel: (636) 220-6334 | Fax: (636) 220-6332

Forest Park Hospital Rehabilitation Services
6150 Oakland Avenue | St. Louis, MO 63139
Tel: (314) 768-3032 | Fax: (314) 768-5654

Harry S. Truman Memorial Veteran's Hospital
800 Hospital Drive | Columbia, MO 65201-5297
Tel: (573) 814-6000 | Fax: (573) 814-6600

Rusk Rehabilitation Center
315 Business Loop 70 West | Columbia, MO 65203 | Fax: (573) 817-4702

St. Francis Medical Center - Center for Health & Wellness Outpatient
Rehab
150 S Mount Auburn | Cape Girardeau, MO 63701 | Tel: (573) 331-5153

Saint Louis University Hospital Geriatric Medicine
3635 Vista Avenue | St. Louis, MO 63110
Tel: (314) 577-8000 | Fax: (314) 577-8003

St. Luke's Hospital Rehabilitation and Medical Center
20 NE Saint Luke's Blvd, Suite 100 | Lee's Summit, MO 64086
Tel: (816) 347-5775

St. Mary's Medical Center - Rehabilitation Services
201 NW R.D. Mize Road | Blue Springs, MO 64014 | Tel: (816) 655-5350

St. Joseph Medical Center - Rehabilitation Services
1000 Carondelet Drive | Kansas City, MO 64114 | Tel: (816) 943-2552

The Rehabilitation Institute of Kansas City
3011 Baltimore | Kansas City, MO 64108
Tel: (816) 751-7729 | Fax: (816) 751-7984

United Access
313 East Ash Street | Columbia, MO 65201
Tel: (888) 939-1010 | Fax: (573) 874-2214

University of Missouri-Columbia, Sinclair School of Nursing Senior Care
Ellis Fischel Cancer Center, DC 900.00, Rm. 2014
115 Business Loop 70W | Columbia, MO 65203 | Tel: (573) 884-2689

Veteran Affairs Medical Center
#1 JB Drive (117/JB) | St. Louis, MO 63125 | Tel: (314) 652-4100

Missouri Driving Regulations

Driver Licensing Agency
Missouri Department of Revenue | Division of Motor Vehicle and Driver
Licensing
Room 470, Truman Office Building | 301 West High Street
Jefferson City, MO 65105 | Tel: (573) 751-4600
Web site: www.dor.state.mo.us

Standard Length of license validation—6 years. Renewal options and
conditions are in person, or renewal by mail if out of state. A vision test is
required at time of renewal and a written and/or road test are required if
license has been expired for more than 6 months (184 days). Also, if an
individual is cited, after the review process a written and/or road test may
be required.

Age-based renewal procedures—At age 70, renewal cycle is reduced to
3 years.

Reporting Procedures

Physician/medical reporting	Reporting is not required. However, for any condition that could impair or limit a person's driving ability, physicians may complete and submit a statement (Form 1528, "Physician's Statement") Form 1528 is available on the Missouri Department of Revenue Web site.
Immunity	Yes, an individual is immune from civil liability when a report is made in good faith.

Legal protection	Medical professionals will not be prevented from making a report because of their physician-patient relationship (302 291 Rsmo).
DMV follow-up	Depending on the information received, the DMV may request additional information; add restrictions; require a written exam, skills test, vision exam, or physical exam; or deny the privilege of driving.
*Other reporting	Will accept information from courts, DMV clerks, peace officers, social workers, and family members within three degrees of consanguinity.
Anonymity	Available

Role of the Medical Advisory Board—The MAB evaluates each case on an individual basis. Action is based on the recommendation of the majority.
Missouri Department of Review | P.O. Box 200
Jefferson City, MO 65105-0200 | Tel: (573) 751-2730

MONTANA

State Office on Aging

Montana Office on Aging Senior and Long Term Care Division
Department of Public Health and Human Services
111 Sanders Street | P.O. Box 4210 | Helena, MT 59604
Tel: (406) 444-7788 | Fax: (406) 444-7743

Driver Rehabilitation and Assessment Programs

Community Medical Center - Occupational Therapy / Driver Evaluation
2827 Fort Missoula Road | Missoula, MT 59804
Tel: (406) 728-4100 | Fax: (406) 327-4580

North Valley Hospital - Rehabilitation Services
6575 Highway 93 South | Whitefish, MT 59937
Tel: (406) 863-3500 | Toll Free: (888) 815-5528 | Fax: (406) 862-2532

Northern Montana Health Care - Just for Seniors
30 13th Street | Havre, MT 59501 | Tel: (406) 265-2211

Research and Training Center on Rural Rehabilitation Services
The University of Montana Rural Institute:
A Center of Excellence in Disabilities Education, Research and Services
52 Corbin Hall | Missoula, MT 59812-7056
Tel: (888) 268-2743 or (406) 243-2654

Rocky Mountain Traffic School Driver Rehabilitation Program
P.O. Box 825 | Livingston, MT 59047
Tel: (406) 686-4968 | Fax: (406) 686-4836

Vocational Rehabilitation/Blind and Low Vision Services
Montana Department of Public Health and Human Services
111 Sanders Street | P. O. Box 4210 | Helena, MT 59604-4210
Tel: (406) 444-2590

Montana Driving Regulations

Driver Licensing Agency
Montana Department of Justice | Motor Vehicle Division
Scott Hart Building, Second Floor | 303 North Roberts
P.O. Box 201460 | Helena, MT 59620-1430
Tel: (406) 444-1773 | Web site: www.doj.state.mt.us

Standard Length of license validation—8 years. If renewing by mail, a
4-year license is issued and the next renewal requires a personal appear-
ance by the applicant. A vision test is required. A written and road test is
only required at the discretion of the examiner if safe operation of the
motor vehicle is in question.

Age-based renewal procedures—Between ages 68–74, all issued/renewed
licenses expire on the client's 75th birthday. At age 75, renewal cycle is
reduced to 4 years.

Reporting Procedures
   Physician/medical reporting   Physicians are encouraged to report.
   Immunity   There is a statute granting physicians
       immunity from liability for reporting in

good faith any patient whom the
physician diagnoses as having a
condition that will significantly impair
the patient's ability to safely operate a
motor vehicle.

Legal protection   N/A
DMV follow-up   N/A

Other reporting   Will accept information from courts,
                           other DMVs, police, family members,
                           and other sources.

Anonymity   Not anonymous or confidential. If
                           requested, the state is required to
                           disclose to the driver the name of the
                           reporter.

Role of the Medical Advisory Board—Montana does not retain a medical
advisory board.

NEBRASKA

State Office on Aging

Nebraska Division of Aging and Disability Services
Department of Health & Human Services | P.O. Box 95044
301 Centennial Mall – South | Lincoln, NE 68509
Tel: (402) 471-2307 | Fax: (402) 471-4619

Driver Rehabilitation and Assessment Programs

Alegent Health Immanuel Rehabilitation Center - Driver Rehabilitation
Program
6901 North 72nd Street | Omaha, NE 68812 | Tel: (402) 572-2275

Center for Independent Living Driver's Training Program
3204 College Street | Grand Foland, NE 68803
Tel: (308) 382-9255 | Fax: (308) 384-7832

Creighton University Medical Center
Occupational Therapy – Pre-Driving Skills Assessments
601 N 30th Street | Omaha, NE 68131
Tel: (402) 449-4248 | Fax: (402) 449-5852

Great Plains Sports and Therapy Center
1115 South Cottonwood | North Platte, NE 69101 | Tel: (402) 481-3777

Madonna Rehabilitation Driver Retraining Program
5401 South St. | Lincoln, NE 68506
Tel: (402) 483-9497 | Toll Free: (800) 676-5448

Methodist Hospital Geriatric Evaluation and Management Clinic
8303 Dodge St. | Omaha, NE 68114
Tel: (402) 354-3152 | Fax: (402) 354-8720

Saint Elizabeth Regional Medical Center - Rehabilitation Services
555 South 70th Street | Lincoln, NE 68510 | Tel: (402) 219-7498

The Nebraska Medical Center Memory Disorders Clinic
S 42nd St & Dewey Ave | Omaha, NE 68131 | Toll Free: (800) 922-0000

University of Nebraska, Kearney - Nebraska Safety Center
West Center Bldg. | Kearney, NE 68849
Tel: (308) 865-8256 | Fax: (308) 865-8257

Nebraska Driving Regulations

Driver Licensing Agency
Nebraska Department of Motor Vehicles | Nebraska State Office
Building
301 Centennial Mall South | P.O. Box 94789 | Lincoln, NE 68509-4789
Tel: (402) 471-2281 | Web site: www.dmv.state.ne.us

Standard Length of license validation—5 years. Renewal options and
conditions are in person. Individuals who are out of state during their
renewal period may renew via mail. A vision test is required at time of
renewal. A written and road test are required only if license has been
expired over 1 year or license is suspended, revoked, or canceled.

Age-based renewal procedures—None

Reporting Procedures
  Physician/medical reporting   Reporting is encouraged but not
                                   required.

Immunity	No
Legal protection	No
DMV *follow-up*	The driver is notified by certified mail that he/she must appear for retesting. The driver is also required to submit a vision and medical statement completed by his/her physician(s) within the past 90 days.
*Other reporting	Will accept information from law enforcement officers and other concerned parties.
Anonymity	Not anonymous. However, the reporter's identity remains confidential unless the driver appeals the denial or cancellation of his/her license in District Court.

Role of the Medical Advisory Board—The MAB advises the DMV concerning the physical and mental ability of an applicant or holder of an operator's license to operate a motor vehicle.

Nebraska Department of Motor Vehicles | 301 Centennial Mall South P.O. Box 94789 | Lincoln, NE 68509

NEVADA

State Office on Aging

Nevada Division for Aging Services - Department of Human Resources
3416 Goni Road, Building D-132 | Carson City, NV 89706
Tel: (775) 687-4210 | Fax: (775) 687-4264

Driver Rehabilitation and Assessment Programs

Adaptive Driving Rehabilitation
5552 Singing Hills Drive | Las Vegas, NV 89130
Tel: (702) 497-3250 | Fax: (702) 259-6624

CareMeridain Las Vegas - People*first* Rehabilitation
7690 Carmen Blvd. | Las Vegas, NV 89128

North Vista Hospital - People*first* Rehabilitation
1409 East Lake Mead Blvd. | North Las Vegas, NV 89030

Red Rock Behavioral Health Hospital - People*first* Rehabilitation
5975 West Twain Avenue | Las Vegas, NV 89103

St. Mary's Personal Assistance Service Program
745 West Moana Lane, Suite 100 | Reno, NV 89509
Tel: (775) 770-3300 | Fax: (775) 770-7708
6375 West Charleston Blvd. | Bldg. WCL, Suite L-200 Room 180
Las Vegas, NV 89146 | Tel: (702) 315-4336 | Fax: (702) 315-4361

St. Rose Dominican Hospitals
Rose de Lima Campus
102 E Lake Mead Parkway | Henderson, NV 89015
Tel: (702) 616-4576
Siena Campus
3001 St. Rose Parkway | Henderson, NV 89052
Tel: (702) 616-5000 | Fax: (702) 616-5576

Torrey Pines Care Center - People*first* Rehabilitation
1701 South Torrey Pines Drive | Las Vegas, NV 89102

University Medical Center Rehabilitation Center
1800 W Charleston Blvd. | Las Vegas, NV 89102
Tel: (702) 383-2239 or (702) 383-2313

Nevada Driving Regulations

Driver Licensing Agency
Nevada Department of Motor Vehicles | 555 Wright Way
Carson City, NV 89711 | Tel: (702) 486-4368, (775) 684-4368 or
(877) 368-7828 Web site: www.dmvnv.com

Standard Length of license validation - 4 years. Renewal options and
conditions are mail-in every other cycle. A vision test is required. A
written and road test is not required, unless license classification has
changed.

Age-based renewal procedures—At age 70, a vision test and medical report are required for mail-in renewal.

Reporting Procedures

Physician/medical reporting	Physicians are required to report patients diagnosed with epilepsy, any seizure disorder, or any other disorder characterized by lapse of consciousness.
Immunity	Yes
Legal protection	Yes
DMV follow-up	The DMV notifies the driver by mail and may suspend his/her license.
*Other reporting	Will accept information from courts, other DMVs, police, and family members.
Anonymity	Available

Role of the Medical Advisory Board—The MAB advises the DMV in the development of medical and health standards for licensure. It also advises the DMV on medical reports submitted regarding the mental or physical condition of individual applicants. The department has the authority to convene a medical advisory board, as stated in Nevada Administrative Code 483.380. However, due to budget constraints, Nevada does not have an advisory board at present.

NEW HAMPSHIRE

State Office on Aging

New Hampshire Bureau of Elderly and Adult Services
Brown Building | 129 Pleasant St. | Concord, NH 03301-3857
Tel: (603) 271-4394 | Fax: (603) 271-4643

Driver Rehabilitation and Assessment Programs

Crotched Mountain Rehabilitation Center
1 Verney Drive | Greenfield, NH 03047
Tel: (603) 547-3311 x292 | Web site: www.cmf.org

HEALTHSOUTH Rehabilitation Hospital Outpatient Center
254 Pleasant Street | Concord, NH 03301 | Tel: (603) 226-9800
Exeter Health Care, Inc. - Drive Ability Program
4 Alumni Drive | Exeter, NH 03833
Fax: (603) 580-7931 | Web site: www.foreveryday.com

Farnum Rehabilitation Center
580 Court Street | Keene, NH 03431 | Tel: (123) 456-7890

Lakes Region General Hospital - Rehabilitation Services
73 Daniel Webster Highway | Belmont, NH | Tel: (603) 524-2852

Northeast Rehabilitation Hospital
70 Butler Street |Salem, NH 03079 | Tel: (603) 893-2900

New Hampshire Driving Regulations

Driver Licensing Agency
New Hampshire Department of Safety | Division of Motor Vehicles
James A. Hayes Building | 10 Hazen Drive | Concord, NH 03305-0002
Tel: (603) 271-2251 | Web site: www.state.nh.us/dmv

Standard Length of license validation—5 years. A vision test is required at time of renewal. There is no written or road test for renewal.

Age-based renewal procedures—At age 75, road test is required with renewal.

Reporting Procedures

Physician/medical reporting	Physicians are encouraged to report.
Immunity	N/A
Legal protection	Not available, as reporting is not a requirement.
DMV follow-up	Full reexamination and, in some cases, an administrative hearing
*Other reporting	Will accept information from courts, other DMVs, police, and family members.
Anonymity	Not anonymous or confidential

Role of the Medical Advisory Board—New Hampshire does not retain a medical advisory board.

NEW JERSEY

State Office on Aging

New Jersey Division of Aging & Community Services
Department of Health & Senior Services
240 W State Street | P.O. Box 807 | Trenton, NJ 08625-0807
Tel: (609) 292-4027 | Fax: (609) 943-3343

Driver Rehabilitation and Assessment Programs

Atlantic Rehabilitation Institute Driver Assessment
Overlook Hospital - Outpatient
99 Beauvoir Avenue | Summit, NJ 07902 | Tel: (908) 522-2000
Mountainside Hospital - Outpatient
Bay & Highland Avenues | Montclair/Glen Ridge, NJ
Tel: (973) 429-6000

Bacharach Institute of Rehabilitation
61 West Jim Leeds Road | Pomona, NJ 08240-0723
Tel: (609) 748-6866 | Fax: (609) 652-9581

Hackensack University Medical Center Division of Geriatrics/Geriatrics
Clinic
30 Prospect Avenue | Hackensack, NJ 07601
Tel: (201) 996-2503 | Fax: (201) 883-0870

Hasbrouck Heights Community Health Center Geriatrics Clinic
212 Terrace Avenue | Hasbrouck Heights, NJ 07604
Tel: (201) 393-7464

HEALTHSOUTH Rehabilitation Center of Toms River
1451 Rt 37 W | Toms River, NJ 08755
Tel: (732) 818-3600 | Fax: (732) 341-0316

Hunterdon Healthcare System, Senior Services - Geriatric Assessment
2100 Wescott Drive | Flemington, NJ 08822 | Tel: (908) 788-6373

JFK Johnson Rehabilitation Institute - Solaris Health System
65 James Street | Edison, NJ 08818
Tel: (732) 321-7056 | Fax: (732) 205-1463

Kessler Institute of Rehabilitation
1199 Pleasant Valley Way | West Orange, NJ 07052
Tel: (973) 731-3900 x2322 | Fax: (973) 243-6842
Web site: www.kessler-rehab.com

Marlton Rehabilitation Hospital Pre-Driver's Screens
92 Brick Rd. | Marlton, NJ 08053 | Tel: (856) 988-8778

Meridian Institute for Aging
1043 Route 70 West, Unit C3 | Manchester Plaza
Lakehurst, NJ 08733 | Tel: (732) 657-6100 | Fax: (732) 657-0111

Newark Beth Israel Medical Center - The Center for Geriatric Health Care
201 Lyons Avenue at Osborne Terrace | Newark, NJ 07112
Tel: (973) 926-7000

Our Lady of Lourdes Medical Center - Lourdes Rehabilitation Center
1600 Haddon Avenue | Camden, NJ 08103 | Tel: (856) 757-3877

Robert Wood Johnson University Hospital - Rehabilitation Services
One Robert Wood Johnson Place | New Brunswick, NJ 08903
Tel: (732) 937-8623

St. Lawrence Rehabilitation Center
2381 Lawrenceville Rd. | Lawrenceville, NJ 08648
Tel: (609) 896-9500 x2494 | Fax: (609) 896-9698

St. Peter's University Hospital
Geriatric Evaluation and Management | Tel: (732) 745-6655
Senior Health Center | Pondview Plaza | 300 Overlook Drive
Monroe Township, NJ 08831 | Tel: (609) 409-1363

The University Hospital, Rehabilitation Therapy Services - Occupational
Therapy
150 Bergen Street, D209 | Newark, NJ 07103 | Tel: (973) 972-4300

New Jersey Driving Regulations

Driver Licensing Agency
New Jersey Motor Vehicle Commission | P.O. Box 160
Trenton, NJ 08666 | Tel: (609) 292-6500 | Web site: www.state.nj.us/mvs

Standard Length of license validation—4 years. Renewal options and
conditions are in person. A vision test may be required at time of renewal.
If recommended by the examiner, a written or road test may be required.

Age-based renewal procedures—None

Reporting Procedures

Physician/medical reporting	Physicians are required to report drivers who experience recurrent loss of consciousness.
Immunity	Yes
Legal protection	No
DMV follow-up	The driver is notified in writing of the referral. There is a scheduled suspension of the license, but the driver may request due process in an administrative court.
Other reporting	Will accept signed letter from police, family, other DMVs, and courts.
Anonymity	Not available

Role of the Medical Advisory Board—The Motor Vehicle Commission
supplies forms for each type of medical condition that may be a cause for
concern. These forms must be completed by the driver's physician.
Problem cases are referred to the MAB, which then makes licensing
recommendations based on the information provided.
New Jersey Motor Vehicle Commission, Medical Division
P.O. Box 173 | Trenton, NJ 08666 | Tel: (609) 292-4035

NEW MEXICO

State Office on Aging

New Mexico Aging & LTC Services Department
2550 Cerrillos Road | Santa Fe, NM 87505
Tel: (505) 476-4799 or (505) 476-4738 | Fax: (505) 827-7649

Driver Rehabilitation and Assessment Programs

Adaptability School of Driving
2716 Vassar Pl., NE | Albuquerque, NM 87107
Tel: (505) 884-8018 | Fax: (505) 884-8007

Independent Mobility Systems
4100 W Piedras Street | Farmington, NM 87401 | Tel: (505) 326-4538

Lea Regional Medical Center - Rehabilitation Therapies
5419 N Lovington Highway | Hobbs, NM 88240 | Tel: (505) 492-5000

Memorial Medical Center - Rehabilitation Services
2450 Telshor Blvd. | Las Cruces, NM 88011 | Tel: (505) 522-8641

New Mexico VA Health Care System
1501 San Pedro Drive SE | Albuquerque, NM 87108-5153
Tel: (505) 265-1711 | Fax: (505) 256-2855

Presbyterian Health Services
Street Address: 2501 Buena Vista SE | Albuquerque, NM
Mailing Address: P.O. Box 26666 | Albuquerque, NM 87125-6666
Arthritis Center: Tel: (505) 823-8321
Rehabilitation Services: Tel: (505) 823-8350 or (505) 291-2372

Rehabilitation Hospital of New Mexico
505 Elm Street NE | Tel: (505) 724-4700

Rehoboth McKinley Christian Hospital - Rehabilitation Services
1901 Red Rock Drive | Gallup, NM 87301 | Tel: (505) 863-7000

San Juan Regional Medical Center - Therapy/Rehabilitation
801 West Maple | Farmington, NM 87401 |Tel: (505) 325-5011

New Mexico Driving Regulations

Driver Licensing Agency
Motor Vehicle Division | New Mexico Taxation and Revenue Department
Joseph Montoya Building | P.O. Box 1028 | Santa Fe, NM 87504-7028
Tel: (888) 683-4636 | Web site: www.state.nm.us

Standard Length of license validation—4 or 8 years. A vision test is required at time of renewal, and written and road tests may be required.

Age-based renewal procedures—Drivers may not apply for 8-year renewal if they will turn 75 during the last 4 years of the 8-year period. At age 75, the renewal interval decreases to 1 year.

Reporting Procedures

Physician/medical reporting	Yes (not specified)
Immunity	Yes
Legal protection	Yes
DMV follow-up	Driver is informed by mail that his/her license will be cancelled in 30 days unless he/she submits a medical report stating that he/she is medically fit to drive.
*Other reporting	Will accept information from courts, other DMVs, police, and family members.
Anonymity	Not anonymous or confidential.

Role of the Medical Advisory Board—The MAB reviews the periodic medical updates that are required for drivers with specific medical conditions (e.g., epilepsy, diabetes, certain heart conditions). The DMV learns of these conditions through questions asked on the application. Tel: (505) 827-2241

NEW YORK

State Office on Aging

New York Office for The Aging
Two Empire State Plaza | Albany, NY 12223-1251
Tel: (518) 474-7012 | Fax: (518) 474-1398

Driver Rehabilitation and Assessment Programs

Access Unlimited
570 Hance Rd. | Binghamton, NY 13903 | Tel: (607) 669-4822

Cognitive and Driver Rehab Services
38-25 52nd Street | Sunnyside, NY 11104
Tel: (718) 457-7483 | Fax: (718) 457-7483
Web site: www.cogrehab.com

Dr. Susan Smith McKinney Nursing and Rehabilitation Center
594 Albany Avenue | Brooklyn, NY 11203 | Tel: (718) 245-7000

Driver Rehabilitation of the Hudson Valley, LLC
110 Main Street, Suite 2E | Poughkeepsie, NY 12601
Tel: (845) 454-4336 | Fax: (845) 452-6871

Erie County Medical Center - Occupational Therapy Department
462 Grider Street | Buffalo, NY 14215
Tel: (716) 898-3235 | Fax: (716) 989-3259

Fitzgerald's Driving School
1350 Deer Park Avenue | North Babylon, NY 11703
Tel: (631) 667-9642 | Fax: (516) 667-8261

Geneva General Hospital Garnsey Rehabilitation Center
196 North Street | Geneva, NY 14456
Tel: (315) 787-5444 | Fax: (315) 787-4573

Hartman Hand and Occupational Therapy
1168 Ridge Crest Drive | Victor, NY 14564
Tel: (315) 462-2569 | Fax: (315) 462-2730

Helen Hayes Hospital
Route 9W | W Haverstraw, NY 10994
Tel. (845) 786-4487 | Fax: (845) 786-4022
Web site: www.helenhayeshosp.org

Meltzer's Driver Training Center
44 Dorothy Heights | Wappingers Falls, NY 12590-3008
Tel: (845) 297-3966 | Fax: (845) 371-3305
Web site: www.drivingAcar.com

New York Presbyterian Hospital
525 East 68th Street, F18 Box 142 | New York, NY 10021 | Tel: (212) 746-1517
Cornell Aging | Tel: (212) 746-7000

Rehab Technology Associates, Inc.
P.O. Box 540 | Kinderhook, NY 12106
Tel: (518) 758-7887 | Fax: (518) 758-8505
Web site: www.retech2000.com

Rochester Rehabilitation Center
1000 Elmwood Ave. | Rochester, NY 14620 | Tel: (585) 271-2520 x716

Schuyler Hospital - Rehabilitation Services
220 Steuben Street | Montour Falls, NY 14865 | Tel: (607) 535-7121
x2206

Staten Island University Hospital Geriatric Consultation Center
450 Seaview Avenue | Tel: (718) 226-8910
Geriatrics Center–South Site
375 Seguine Avenue | Tel: (718) 226-2515
Geriatrics Center–North Site
242 Mason Avenue | Tel: (718) 226-6323 or (718) 226-6322

Sunnyview Rehabilitation Hospital - Driver Re-Training
128 Bruce Street | Scotia, NY 12302

The Burke Rehabilitation Hospital - Driver Evaluation Program
785 Mamaroneck Avenue | White Plains, NY 10605 | Tel: (914) 597-2326

The Rusk Institute of Rehabilitation Medicine – Outpatient Services
New York University Hospitals Center - Rusk Institute
550 First Avenue | New York, NY 10016 | Tel: (212) 263-6037

Transitions of Long Island
1554 Northern Blvd. | Manhasset, NY 11030
Tel: (516) 719-3700 | Fax: (516) 365-4748

New York Driving Regulations

Driver Licensing Agency
New York State Department of Motor Vehicles | 6 Empire State Plaza
Albany, NY 12228 | Tel: (212) 645-5550, (800) 342-5368, or (800) 225-5368
Web site: www.nydmv.state.ny.us

Standard Length of license validation—First time renewal is 4 years, then
every 8 years. Renewal options and conditions are in person or mail-in. A
vision test is required at time of renewal and clients must pass a vision test
at the DMV office or submit Form MV-619. A written or road test is not
required.

Age-based renewal procedures—None

Reporting Procedures

Physician/medical reporting	Permitted but not required
Immunity	No
Legal protection	N/A
DMV follow-up	If a physician reports a condition that can affect the driving skills of a patient, the DMV may suspend the driver's license until a physician provides certification that the condition has been treated or controlled and no longer affects driving skills. If the DMV receives a report from a source that is not a physician, the DMV considers each case individually.
*Other reporting	Will accept information from courts, other DMVs, police, family members,

and other sources. Letters must be signed.

Anonymity   Not anonymous. Also, if a person in a professional or official position (i.e., physician) reports, the DMV will disclose the identity of the reporter; however, if the reporter does not fall under this category, the identity of the reporter is protected under the Freedom of Information Law.

Role of the Medical Advisory Board—The MAB advises the commissioner on medical criteria and vision standards for the licensing of drivers. New York State Department of Motor Vehicles | Medical Review Unit Room 220 | 6 Empire State Plaza | Albany, NY 12228-0220

NORTH CAROLINA

State Office on Aging

North Carolina Division of Aging & Adult Services
Department of Health and Human Services
2101 Mail Service Center | 693 Palmer Drive | Raleigh, NC 27699-2101
Tel: (919) 733-3983 | Fax: (919) 733-0443

Driver Rehabilitation and Assessment Programs

Bryant Driving School
Durham/Chapel Hill Tel: (919) 489-7550 | Raleigh Tel: (919) 782-3266

Cape Fear Valley Health System
Southeastern Regional Rehabilitation Center
1638 Owen Dr. | Fayetteville, NC 28304 | Tel: (910) 609-4000

Carolinas Driving School for the Disabled
Toll Free: (800) 634-2256

Charlotte Institute of Rehabilitation
1100 Blythe Boulevard | Charlotte, NC 28120
Tel: (704) 355-0779 | Fax: (704) 355-5987

Coastal Rehabilitation Hospital
2131 S 17th Street | Wilmington, NC 28401 | Tel: (910) 343-7845

Driver Rehabilitation Services
1200 St. Joseph St., #63 | Carolina Beach, NC 28428
Tel: (910) 763-8184 | Fax: (336) 697-7842
Web site: www.driver-rehabnc.com

Duke University Health System - Occupational Therapy
Clinical Driving Evaluation/Driver Preparation
Lenox Baker Hospital | 3000 Erwin Road | Durham, NC
Tel: (919) 684-4543 | Fax: (919) 668-2420

First Health of the Carolinas - Occupational Therapy Department
P.O. Box 3000 | Driver Rehabilitation Program | Pinehurst, NC 28374
Tel: (910) 215-1637 | Fax: (910) 215-1665

Frye Regional Medical Center
420 North Center Street | Hickory, NC 28601
Tel: (828) 315-3712 | Fax: (828) 315-5587

Independence Rehabilitation Center
2800 Ashton Drive, Suite B | Wilmington, NC 28412
Tel: (910) 342-3270 | Fax: (910) 332-0129

Moses Cone Outpatient Rehab
1904 N Church Street | Greensboro, NC 27405 | Tel: (336) 271-4840

Oleander Rehabilitation Center
5220 Oleander Drive | Wilmington, NC 28401
Tel: (910) 452-8104 | Fax: (910) 452-8666

Regional Rehabilitation Center - Outpatient Rehabilitation Center
University Health Systems of Eastern Carolina - InRoads Driving
Evaluation
2310 Stantonsburg Road | Tel: (252) 847-6600

The Rehabilitation Center at UNC Hospitals
NC Memorial Hospital, 7th Floor | 101 Manning Drive
Chapel Hill, NC, 27599 | Tel: (919) 966-5666

Thoms Rehabilitation Hospital, Outpatient Center - Driver's Evaluation
68 Sweeten Creek Road | Asheville, NC 28803
Tel. (828) 274-6179 | Fax: (828) 277-4841

University of North Carolina Program on Aging
141 MacNider Building | Campus Box 7550
Chapel Hill, NC 27599-7550 | Tel: (919) 966-5945

Wake Forest University Baptist Medical Center - Adaptive Driving
Program
Comprehensive Rehabilitation Plaza | 131 Miller Street
Winston-Salem, NC 27103 | Tel: (336) 716-8004 | Fax: (336) 716-8005

North Carolina Driving Regulations

Driver Licensing Agency
North Carolina Department of Transportation | Division of Motor Vehicles
1100 New Bern Avenue | Raleigh, NC 27698 | Tel: (919) 715-7000
Web site: www.dmv.dot.state.nc.us

Standard Length of license validation—5 years. Renewal options and
conditions are in person. A vision and written test are required, but a road
test is not.

Age-based renewal procedures—Drivers age 60 and older are not required
to parallel park on their road test.

Reporting Procedures

Physician/medical reporting	Physicians are encouraged to report unsafe drivers.
Immunity	North Carolina statutes protect the physician who reports an unsafe driver.
Legal protection	No
DMV follow-up	Driver is notified in writing of referral.
*Other reporting	Will accept information from courts, other DMVs, police, family members, and other sources. Letters must be signed.

Anonymity	Not anonymous or confidential. The driver may request a copy of his/her records.

Role of the Medical Advisory Board—The MAB reviews all medical information that is submitted to the DMV and determines what action should be taken. These actions can be appealed.
North Carolina Division of Motor Vehicles | Medical Review Unit
3112 Mail Service Center | Raleigh, NC 27697
Tel: (919) 861-3809 | Fax: (919) 733-9569

NORTH DAKOTA

State Office on Aging

North Dakota Aging Services Division - Department of Human Services
600 East Boulevard Avenue | Department 325 | Bismarck, ND 58505-0250
Tel: (701) 328-4601 | Fax: (701) 328-2359

Driver Rehabilitation and Assessment Programs

Great Plains Rehabilitation Services
1212 East Main Avenue | Bismark, ND 58501
Tel: (701) 530-4000 | Toll free: (800) 222-4989 | Fax: (701) 530-4001

Heart of America Medical Center Outpatient Wellness – Occupational Therapy
800 South Main Avenue | Rugby, ND 58368-2198 | Tel: (701) 776-5261

MedCenter One
300 N 7th Street | P.O. Box 5525 | Bismarck, ND 58506-5525
Tel: (701) 323-6544 | Fax: (701) 323-6189
Web site: www.medcenterone.com

Mercy Medical Center - Rehabilitation Services
1301 15th Avenue West | Williston, ND 58801 | Tel: (701) 774-7436

Merit Care Hospital - Occupational Therapy Department
1720 S University Dr. | Fargo, ND 58103
Tel: (701) 280-4070 | Fax: (701) 280-4419

Merit Care Medical Center
OT Driving Dept., #306 | 720 4th Street North | Fargo, ND 58122
Tel: (701) 280-4078 | Fax: (701) 280-1419

Meithcare Hospital – Occupational Therapy Department
720 Fourth Street N | Fargo, ND 58122
Tel: (701) 280-4070 | Fax: (701) 234-7451

St. Alexius Balance and Dizziness Center - Human Performance Center
310 N 9th Street | Bismark, ND 58501
Tel: (701) 530-8106 | Toll Free: (800) 222-7858

St. Aloisius Medical Center - Occupational Therapy
325 East Brewster Street | Harvey, ND 58341
Tel: (701) 324-4651 | Fax: (701) 324-4651

St. Joseph's Hospital & Health Center - Rehabilitation Services
30 West Seventh Street | Dickinson, ND 58601
Tel: (701) 456-4000 | Fax: (701) 456-4829

Tip Top Mobility, Inc.
6 Stemen Drive | Burlington, ND 58722
Toll Free: (800) 735-5958

North Dakota Driving Regulations

Driver Licensing Agency
North Dakota Department of Transportation
Drivers License and Traffic Safety Division | 608 East Boulevard
Bismarck, ND 58505-0700 | Tel: (701) 328-2600
Web site: www.state.nd.us/dot

Standard Length of license validation—4 years. A vision test is required at time of renewal, however, written and road tests are not.

Age-based renewal procedures—None

Reporting Procedures
  Physician/medical reporting   Physicians are permitted by law to
                                     report to the Drivers License and

	Traffic Safety Division in writing the name, date of birth, and address of any patient over the age of 14 whom they have reasonable cause to believe is incapable, due to physical or mental reason, of safely operating a motor vehicle.
Immunity	Physicians who in good faith make a report, give an opinion, make a recommendation, or participate in any proceeding pursuant to this law are immune from liability.
Legal protection	Available. North Dakota Century Code addresses medical advice provided by physicians.
DMV follow-up	Vision and/or medical reports may be required.
Other reporting	Will accept information from courts, other DMVs, police, and family members.
Anonymity	Not available

Role of the Medical Advisory Board—The MAB participates in drafting administrative rules for licensing standards. Tel: (701) 328-2070

OHIO

State Office on Aging

Ohio Department of Aging
50 West Broad Street, 9th Floor | Columbus, OH 43215-5928
Tel: (614) 466-7246 | Fax: (614) 995-1049

Driver Rehabilitation and Assessment Programs

Capabilities, Inc.
124 S Front Street | Saint Marys, OH 45885
Tel: (419) 394-0003 | Fax: (419) 394-2853

Cleveland Clinic Foundation
4294 Oviatt Road | Cleveland, OH 44195 | Tel: (216) 445-8479

Coghlin Rehabilitation Center - MUO Outpatient Rehabilitation Services
Driving Assessment and Training
3065 Arlington Avenue | Toledo, OH 43614
Tel: (419) 383-5040 | Toll free: (800) 321-8383 x5040 | Fax: (419) 383-3184

Cuyahoga Falls General Hospital Natatorium Rehabilitation and Wellness
Center
2345 4th Street | Cuyahoga Falls, OH 44221 | Tel: (330) 926-0384

D & D Driving Schools, Inc.
3125 Wilmington Pike | Kettering, OH 45429
Tel: (937) 294-7206 | Fax: (937) 290-0696
Web site: www.dnddrivingschools.com

Drive Ways Driving School
1229 Lincoln Highway | P.O. Box 613 | Van Wert, OH 45891
Tel: (419) 238-1496

Edwin Shaw Hospital - Occupational Therapy Department
1621 Flickinger Rd. | Akron, OH 44312
Tel: (330) 650-9610 | Fax: (330) 733-2975
Web site: www.edinshaw.com

Forward Motions, Inc.
214 Valley Street | Dayton, OH 45404 | Tel: (937) 222-5001

Grady Memorial Hospital - Rehabilitation Services
561 W Central Avenue | Delaware, OH 43015
Tel: (740) 368-5002 | Fax: (740) 368-5003

Heights Driving School
5241 Wilson Mills Road | Richmond Heights, OH 44143
Tel: (440) 449-3300 | Web site: www.heightsdriving.com

Hillside Rehabilitation Hospital Driver Evaluation and Training
8747 Squires Lane NE | Warren, OH 44484 | Tel: (330) 841-3700

Key Mobility Services
1944 U.S. State Route 68 N | Xenia, OH 45385 | Tel: (937) 427-1323

Marietta Memorial Hospital
401 Matthew Street | Marietta, OH 45750
Tel: (740) 374-1438 | Web site: www.mmhospital.org

Medical College of Ohio Driver Rehabilitation Program
Tel: (419) 861-4458

Mercy Medical Center–Driving School
1320 Mercy Drive NW | Canton, OH 44708
Tel: (330) 489-1135 | Fax: (330) 430-6972

MetroHealth Driver Rehabilitation Program
4310 Richmond Rd. | Highland Hills, OH 44122 | Tel: (216) 595-7890

Miami Valley Hospital
One Wyoming Street | Dayton, OH 45459 | Tel: (937) 208-4181

MobilityWorks
810 Moe Drive | Akron, OH 44310 | Tel: (330) 633-1118

Mount Carmel Senior Services Memory Disorders Clinic | Tel: (614) 234-8170
Mount Carmel East | 6001 East Broad Street | Tel: (614) 234-6077
Mount Carmel West | 730 West Rich Street | Tel: (614) 234-8170

North West Ohio Driver Training School, Inc.
101 S Defiance St., Box 26 | Stryker, OH 43557
Tel: (419) 682-4741 | Fax: (419) 682-4742

OhioHealth Rehabilitation Center
4664 Larwell Drive | Columbus, OH 43220
Tel: (614) 566-1120 | Fax: (614) 566-1130

Ohio Safe-T-Brake, Inc.
1137 Market Avenue N | Canton, OH 44702 | Toll Free: (800) 773-4104

Ohio State University Medical Center
2050 Kenny Rd. | Columbus, OH 43221
Tel: (740) 862-6594 | Fax: (614) 293-5220

Summa Fall Prevention and Balance Program, St. Thomas Hospital
444 N Main St. | Akron, OH | Tel: (330) 379-5170

Total Rehab at Flower Hospital
5150 Harroun Road | Sylvania, OH 43560
Tel: (419) 824-1968 | Fax: (419) 824-1773

Vision Center of Central Ohio, Inc.
1393 N High Street | Columbus, OH 43201 | Tel: (614) 294-5571

Ohio Driving Regulations

Driver Licensing Agency
Ohio Department of Public Safety | Bureau of Motor Vehicles
P.O. Box 16520 | Columbus, OH 43216-6520 | Tel: (614) 752-7500
Web site: www.state.oh.us/odps

Standard Length of license validation—4 years. Renewal options and
conditions are done in person. Clients may renew by mail only if they
are out of state. A vision test is required, however, written and road tests
are not.

Age-based renewal procedures—None

Reporting Procedures
   Physician/medical reporting   Ohio will accept and act on information submitted by a physician regard-
ing an unsafe driver. The physician
must agree to be a source of information and allow the Bureau of Motor
Vehicles to divulge this information to
the driver.

   Immunity   No
   Legal protection   No
   DMV follow-up   A letter is sent requiring the driver to
submit a medical statement and/or take

a driver's license examination. The driver is given 30 days to comply.

Other reporting

Will accept information from courts, law enforcement agencies, hospitals, rehabilitation facilities, family, and friends.

Anonymity

Not anonymous or confidential

Role of the Medical Advisory Board—Ohio does not have a medical advisory board. The Bureau of Motor Vehicles contacts a medical consultant for assistance with difficult cases or for policy-making assistance.

OKLAHOMA

State Office on Aging

Aging Services Division - OK Department of Human Services
P.O. Box 25352 | 2401 NW 23rd St., Suite 40
Oklahoma City, OK 73107-2413 | Tel: (405) 521-2281 | Fax: (405) 521-2086

Driver Rehabilitation and Assessment Programs

Bone & Joint Hospital
1111 N Dewey Ave. | Oklahoma City, OK 73103 | Tel: (405) 272-9671

Deaconess Hospital Senior Diagnostics Center
5501 North Portland | Oklahoma City, OK 73112 | Tel: (405) 604-6138

Integris Jim Thorpe Rehab Driving Program
603 Okmulgee | Norman, OK 73071
Tel: (405) 644-5423 | Fax: (405) 636-7178

Kaiser Rehab Center
Hillcrest Medical Center | 1125 S Trenton | Tulsa, OK 74120
Tel: (918) 579-7111 | Fax: (918) 579-7110

Midwest Rehab Medicine
1201 S Douglas Blvd., Suite I | Midwest City, OK 73130
Tel: (405) 610-8090

Oklahoma City Veterans Affairs Medical Center
921 NE 13th Street | Oklahoma City, OK 73104
Tel: (405) 270-0501 | Fax: (405) 270-1560

Oklahoma University Medical Center - The Reynolds Geriatric Department
1200 Everett Drive | Oklahoma City, OK 73104 | Tel: (405) 271-4700

Rolling Hills Geriatric Services
1000 Rolling Hills Lane | Ada, OK 74820
Tel: (580) 436-3600 | Crisis Number: (800) 522-9505
Web site: www.rollinghillshospital.com

Simulator Systems International, Inc.
11130 E 56th Street | Tulsa, OK 74146-6713 | Tel: (918) 250-4500

St. Anthony Behavioral Medicine
Geriatric Diagnostic Center/St. Michael Campus
2129 SW 59th Street | Oklahoma City, OK 73119 | Tel: (405) 713-5733

St. Francis Hospital - Broken Arrow Rehabilitation
3000 South Elm Place | Broken Arrow, Oklahoma 74012
Tel: (918) 455-3535

St. John's Chapman Outpatient Rehabilitation Clinic
Chapman Health Plaza Building | 1819 E 19th Street | Tulsa, OK 74104
Tel: (918) 744-2476 | Fax: (918) 744-3075

St. Mary's Center for Rehabilitation
HealthPlex Center in Willow Plaza
2123 W Willow | Enid, OK 73703
Tel: (580) 237-8278 | Fax (580) 237-7641

Oklahoma Driving Regulations

Driver Licensing Agency
Oklahoma Department of Public Safety | Driver Licensing Services
P.O. Box 11415 | Oklahoma City, OK 73136-0415 | Tel: (405) 425-2059
Web site: www.dps.state.ok.us

Standard Length of license validation—4 years. Renewal options and conditions are done in-person. There are no vision, written, or road tests at time of renewal.

Age-based renewal procedures—License fee reduced for drivers 62–64 years old. Fees waived for 65 and older.

Reporting Procedures

Physician/medical reporting	Physicians are permitted to report to the Department of Public Safety any patient whom they have reasonable cause to believe is incapable of safely operating a motor vehicle.
Immunity	Any physician reporting in good faith and without malicious intent shall have immunity from civil liability that might otherwise be incurred.
Legal protection	By statute the physician has full immunity.
DMV follow-up	The driver is notified in writing of the referral and required to appear for an interview at the Department. The Department also requires a current medical evaluation from a qualified practitioner.
*Other reporting	Will accept information from any verifiable source with direct knowledge of the medical condition that would render a driver unsafe.
Anonymity	Not available

Role of the Medical Advisory Board—The MAB advises the Department of Public Safety on medical issues regarding individual drivers. Actions are based on the recommendation of the majority and/or specialist.
Oklahoma Department of Public Safety | Executive Medical Secretary
P.O. Box 11415 | Oklahoma City, OK 73136-0415

OREGON

State Office on Aging

Oregon Senior & Disabled Services Division - Department of Human Services
500 Summer St. NE, E02 | Salem, OR 97301-1073
Tel: (503) 945-5811 | Fax: (503) 373-7823

Driver Rehabilitation and Assessment Programs

A.B.C. Driving School, Inc.
10450 NW Laidlaw Road | Portland, OR 97229
Tel: (503) 297-1099 | Fax: (503) 292-7211

Adventist Medical Center - Hand and Occupational Rehabilitation
10201 SE Main, Suite 4 | Portland, OR 97216
Tel: (503) 251-6350 | Fax: (503) 251-6846
13435 SE 97th, LL #101 | Clackamas, OR 97015
Tel: (503) 513-7450 | Fax: (503) 513-7449
16096 SE 15th St. | Vancouver, WA 98683
Tel: (360) 882-6894 | Fax: (360) 882-0263

Alpine Rehabilitation & Wellness
4370 NE Halsey St. | Portland, OR 97213
Tel: (503) 249-3220 | Fax: (503) 249-3228

Casey Eye Institute Low Vision Rehabilitation Clinic
3375 SW Terwilliger Blvd. | Portland, OR 97239-4197
Tel: (503) 494-3098

Generations Therapy
Town Center Village | 8611 SE Causey Avenue | Portland, OR 97266
Tel: (503) 654-1939 | Fax: (503) 594-2294

McKenzie-Willamette Medical Center - Rehabilitation Services
1460 G Street | Springfield, OR 97477 | Tel: (541) 744-8474

River Road Physical Therapy Clinic
2401 River Road | Eugene, OR 97404 | Tel: (541) 461-3474

Oregon Driver Education Center, Inc.
1320 Capitol Street NE, Suite 110 |Salem, OR 97303
Tel: (503) 581-3783

O.T. Services: Driving Solutions
1410 Orchard St., Suite 105 | Eugene, OR 97403
Tel: (541) 686-3524 | Fax: (541) 686-2683

Performance Mobility, Inc.
4347 NW Yeon Avenue | Portland, OR 97210 | Tel: (503) 243-2940

Portland Veterans Affairs Medical Center
3710 SW U.S. Veterans Hospital Road | Portland, OR 97239
Tel: (503) 220-8262 | Fax: (503) 273-5319

Senior Health and Wellness Center–Barger Clinic
4010 Aerial Way | Eugene, OR | Tel: (541) 242-8300

St. Charles Hospital—Occupational Therapy
2500 NE Neff Rd. | Bend, OR 97701 | Tel: (541) 617-3987

Oregon Driving Regulations

Driver Licensing Agency
Oregon Department of Transportation | Driver and Motor Vehicle
Services
1905 Lana Avenue NE | Salem, OR 97314 | Tel: (503) 945-5000
Web site: www.odot.state.or.us/dmv

Standard Length of license validation—8 years. Renewal options and
conditions are done by mail-in every other cycle. A vision test is required
at time of renewal only after age 50.

Age-based renewal procedures—After age 50, vision screening is required
every 8 years.

Reporting Procedures
  Physician/medical reporting   Oregon has mandatory medical
                                        impairment-based reporting system.
                                        Physicians and healthcare providers

meeting the definition of "primary care provider" are required to report persons presenting functional and/or cognitive impairments that are severe and cannot be corrected/controlled by surgery, medication, therapy, driving devices, or techniques. The state also has a voluntary reporting system that can be utilized by doctors, law enforcement officers, family, and friends who have concerns about an individual's ability to safely operate a motor vehicle. Reports submitted under the voluntary system may be based on a medical condition or on unsafe driving behaviors exhibited by the individual.

Immunity   Under the mandatory reporting system, primary care providers are exempt from liability for reporting.

Legal protection   Under the mandatory reporting system, the law provides the primary care provider with legal protection for breaking the patient's confidentiality.

DMV follow-up   In most cases, the driving privileges of individuals reported under the mandatory system are immediately suspended. An individual may request the opportunity to demonstrate the ability to safely operate a motor vehicle via knowledge and driving tests. For cognitive impairments (and for specific functional impairments), a medical file and driving record are sent to the State Health Office for determination of whether the individual is safe to drive at the current point in time.

Other reporting   Under the voluntary system, the
                                DMVS will accept information from
                                courts, other DMVs, law enforcement
                                officers, physicians, family members,
                                and other sources.

Anonymity   Reporting is not anonymous. Under
                                the mandatory system, only the
                                medical information being reported is
                                confidential. Under the voluntary
                                system, the DMVS will make every
                                attempt to hold the reporter's name
                                confidential if requested.

Role of the Medical Advisory Board—Oregon does not retain a medical
advisory board. The State Health Office reviews medical cases and makes
licensing decisions by reviewing an individual's medical condition and
ability to drive.
Oregon Driver and Motor Vehicle Services | Driver Programs Section
1905 Lana Avenue NE | Salem, OR 97314 | Tel: (503) 945-5520

PENNSYLVANIA

State Office on Aging

Pennsylvania Department of Aging
555 Walnut Street, 5th Floor | Harrisburg, PA 17101-1919
Tel: (717) 783-1550 | Fax: (717) 772-3382

Driver Rehabilitation and Assessment Programs

Adventist WholeHealth Lifestyle Medicine Center
1025 Berkshire Blvd., Suite 700 | Wyomissing, PA 19610
Tel: (610) 685-9900 | Fax: (610) 685-7171

Brant's Driving School, Inc.
1614 Debran Lane | Johnstown, PA 15905
Tel: (814) 255-3313 | Fax: (814) 255-3313
Web site: www.brantsdrivingschool.com

Bryn Mawr Rehabilitation Hospital
414 Paoli Pike | P.O. Box 3007 | Malvern, PA 19355-3300
Tel: (610) 251-5688 | Fax: (610) 296-4915
Web site: www.brynmawrrehab.org

Butler Veterans Affairs Medical Center - Rehabilitation Department
325 New Castle Road | Butler, PA 16001-2480
Tel: (724) 477-5047 | Toll Free: (800) 362-8262, x5047

CAT/University of Pittsburgh Rehab Science & Technology
SHRS, Suite 5044, Forbes Tower | Pittsburgh, PA 15260
Tel: (412) 647-1312

Center for Assistive & Rehabilitative Technology @ HGAC
727 Goucher Street | Johnstown, PA 15905
Tel: (814) 255-8307 | Fax: (814) 255-8303

Center for Rehabilitation and Sports Medicine
Barclay Square Shopping Center | 1500 Garrett Rd.
Upper Darby, PA 19082 | Tel: (610) 284-8670

Chestnut Hill Rehabilitation Hospital Driver Assessments
SAFE Program (Senior Activity and Functional Evaluation)
8601 Stenton Ave. | Wyndmoor, PA 19038
Tel: (215) 233-6246 | Fax: (215) 233-6339

Crozer-Chester Medical Center Physical & Rehabilitation Medicine
One Medical Center Boulevard | Upland, PA 19013-3995
Tel: (610) 447-2736

Crozer-Keystone Health System Geriatric Evaluation and Management
Program
Tel: (610) 499-7180 | Toll Free: (800) CKHS-KEY or (800) 254-7539

Gettysburg Health Center at Herr's Ridge and Aquatic Center
Driving Evaluations | 820 Chambersburg Road | Gettysburg, PA 17325
Tel: (717) 337-4206

Good Shepherd Rehab Hospital
820 S Fifth Street | Allentown, PA 18018
Tel: (610) 776-8302 | Fax: (610) 776-3551

HEALTHSouth Reading Rehabilitation Hospital—Driver Evaluation
Program
1623 Morgantown Road | Reading, PA 19607
Tel: (610) 796-6480 | Fax: (610) 796-6345

Milton S. Hershey Medical Center Driver—Training/Evaluation
P.O. Box 850 | Mail Code H125 | Hershey, PA 17033
500 University Drive | Hershey, PA 17078 | Tel: (717) 531-7105
Tel: (717) 531-7444 | Fax: (717) 531-0280

John Heinz Institute of Rehabilitation Medicine—Occupational
Therapy
150 Mundy Street | Wilkes-Barre Township, PA 18702
Tel: (570) 826-3895

Keller Handicap Driver Training School
197 Main Street | Luzerne, PA 18709
Tel: (570) 288-1071 | Fax: (570) 288-8070

Magee Rehabilitation Hospital
1513 Race Street | Philadelphia, PA 19102-1177 | Tel: (215) 587-3117

Mercy Fitzgerald Hospital - Sister Marie Lenahan Mercy Wellness Center
1500 Lansdowne Ave. | Darby, PA 19023
PT Tel: (610) 237-4385 | Occupational Therapy Tel: (610) 237-4386
Speech Tel: (610) 237-5688 | Hearing and Balance Tel: (610) 237-4388

Moss Rehabilitation Driving School, Doylestown Hospital
Rehabilitation
Driver / Pre-Driver Screening Program | Einstein Plaza
201 Old York Rd., Suite 203 | Jenkintown, PA 19046-3200
Tel: (215) 886-7706 | Fax: (215) 886-7709
Web site: www.mossresource.net

Nesquehoning Therapy Center
50 East Locust Street | Nesquehoning, PA 18240 | Tel: (570) 669-6580

Penn Forest Therapy Center
Route 903 & Old Stage Road | Albrightsville, PA 18210
Tel: (570) 722-3318

Physical Medicine & Rehabilitation, Springfield Hospital at the Health-plex®
Ground Floor, Pavilion I | 190 West Sproul Rd. | Springfield, PA 19064
Tel: (610) 328-8800

Susquehanna Health System Gibson Rehab Center
777 Rural Avenue | Williamsport, PA 17701
Tel: (717) 321-1000 | Fax: (717) 321-3719

TheraPlex of Nazareth Hospital - Outpatient Therapy Services
8131 Roosevelt Boulevard | Philadelphia, PA | Tel: (215) 335-3954

Transportation Solutions
3837 W 20th Street | Erie, PA 16505
Tel: (814) 833-2301 | Fax: (814) 835-8178 | Web site: www.drivingneeds.com

University of Pennsylvania Medical Center Rehabilitation Hospital
1405 Shady Avenue | Pittsburgh, PA 15217 | Tel: (412) 420-2413

WellSpan Center for Aging
300 Pine Grove Commons | York, PA 17403
Tel: (717) 851-5736 | Toll Free: (888) 603-1540

Wills Eye Low Vision Service
Suite 1010 | 840 Walnut Street | Philadelphia, PA 19107
Tel: (215) 928-3450 | Fax: (215) 928-7234

Pennsylvania Driving Regulations

Driver Licensing Agency
Pennsylvania Department of Transportation | Driver and Vehicle Services
1101 South Front Street | Harrisburg, PA 17104-2516
Tel: (800) 932-4600 or (717) 391-6190 | Web site: www.dot.state.pa.us

Standard Length of license validation—4 years. Renewal options and conditions are available through the Internet, mail, or in person. There are no vision, written or road tests at time of renewal.

Age-based renewal procedures—Drivers aged 65+ renew every 2 years. Drivers aged 45+ are requested to submit a physical and vision exam report prior to renewing (through a random mailing of 1,650 per month).

Reporting Procedures

Physician/medical reporting	"All physicians and other persons authorized to diagnose or treat disorders and disabilities defined by the Medical Advisory Board shall report to PENNDOT in writing the full name, DOB, and address of every person 15 years of age and older, diagnosed as having any specified disorder or disability within 10 days." Physicians must report neuromuscular conditions (e.g., Parkinson's), neuropsychiatric conditions (e.g., Alzheimer's dementia), cardiovascular, cerebrovascular, convulsive, and other conditions that may impair driving ability.
Immunity	"No civil or criminal action may be brought against any person or agency for providing the information required under this system."
Legal protection	Available
DMV follow-up	PENNDOT sends the appropriate correspondence to the driver asking him/her to submit the necessary forms and examination reports.
*Other reporting	Will accept information from courts, other DMVs, police, emergency personnel, family members, neighbors,

and caregivers. Reports must be signed
in order to confirm reporter facts.

Anonymity   Reporting is not anonymous, but the
                                     identity of the reporter will be
                                     protected.

Role of the Medical Advisory Board—The MAB advises PENNDOT and
reviews regulations proposed by PENNDOT concerning physical and
mental criteria (including vision standards) relating to the licensing of
drivers. The MAB meets once every 2 years or as needed.

RHODE ISLAND

State Office on Aging

Rhode Island Department of Elderly Affairs
John O. Pastore Center | Benjamin Rush Building, No. 55
35 Howard Ave. | Cranston, RI 02920
Tel: (401) 462-0500 | Fax: (401) 462-0503

Driver Rehabilitation and Assessment Programs

Atwood Therapy Services
1526 Atwood Avenue, Suite 110 | Johnston, RI 02919
Tel: (401) 621-3281

Easter Seals Rhode Island
5 Woodruff Ave. | Narragansett, RI 02882 | Tel: (401) 284-1000

Landmark Medical Center - Senior Health
176 Cass Ave. | Woonsocket, RI | Tel: (401) 769-4100, x2006

Memorial Hospital of Rhode Island
Alzheimer's Disease & Memory Disorders Center
111 Brewster St. | Pawtucket, RI 02860 | Tel: (401) 729-2483

Rehabilitation Hospital of Rhode Island - Outpatient Services
116 Eddie Dowling Highway | North Smithfield, RI 02896
Tel: (401) 766-0800

Rhode Island Hospital - Alzheimer's Disease and Memory Disorders
Center
6th Floor | 593 Eddy Street | Providence, RI 02903 | Tel: (401) 444-6440

Roger Williams Medical Center - Senior Care
825 Chalkstone Avenue | Providence, RI 02908 | Tel: (405) 456-2000

South County Hospital - Back in Action
53 Spring Street | Peace Dale, RI 2879 | Tel: (401) 792-3503

University Medicine Foundation Geriatrics Practice
407 East Avenue, Suite 110 | Pawtucket, RI 02860 | Tel: (401) 728-7270

Rhode Island Driving Regulations

Driver Licensing Agency
Rhode Island Division of Motor Vehicles | 286 Main Street
Pawtucket, PI 02860
Tel: (401) 588-3020 | Web site: www.dmv.state.ri.us

Standard Length of license validation—5 years. A vision test is required at
time of renewal, however, a written or road test is not required.

Age-based renewal procedures—At age 70, the renewal cycle is reduced to 2
years.

Reporting Procedures
   Physician/medical reporting   Any physician who diagnoses a physical
or mental condition which, in the
physician's judgment, will significantly
impair the person's ability to safely
operate a motor vehicle may voluntarily
report the person's name and other
information relevant to the condition to
the medical advisory board within the
Registry of Motor Vehicles.

   Immunity   Any physician reporting in good faith
and exercising due care shall have
immunity from any liability, civil or
criminal. No cause of

	action may be brought against any physician for not making a report.
Legal protection	N/A
DMV follow-up	Driver is notified in writing of referral.
*Other reporting	Will accept information from courts, other DMVs, police, and family members.
Anonymity	N/A

Role of the Medical Advisory Board—The MAB advises the Division of Motor Vehicles on medical issues regarding individual drivers. Actions are based on the recommendation of the majority.

SOUTH CAROLINA

State Office on Aging

South Carolina Lieutenant Governor's Office on Aging - Bureau of Senior Services
1301 Gervais Street, Suite 200 | Columbia, SC 29201
Tel: (803) 734-9900 | Fax: (803) 734-9886

Driver Rehabilitation and Assessment Programs

Atlantic Physical Therapy & Rehabilitation, Inc.
3650 Coalition Drive | Myrtle Beach, SC 29577
Tel: (843) 293-7713 | Fax: (843) 293-1855

Hilton Head Medical Center Physical Rehabilitation Clinic
24 Bethea Drive | P.O. Box 21117 | Hilton Head Is, SC 29925
Tel: (843) 342-2989 x120 | Fax: (843) 689-6350

Medical University of South Carolina Family Medicine Center
Geriatric Assessment Clinic | 295 Calhoun Street | P.O. Box 250192
Charleston, SC | Tel: 792-1414 | Toll Free: (800) 424-6872

Mobility Unlimited
8410 Rivers Avenue, Suite E | N Charleston, SC 29406
Tel: (843) 797-5700

Roger C. Peace Rehab - Occupational Therapy Department
701 Grove Road | Greenville, SC 29605
Tel: (864) 455-4959 | Fax: (864) 455-7717

Spartanburg Regional Healthcare System - Network Geriatric Services
101 East Wood Street | Spartanburg, SC 29303 | Tel: (864) 542-2756

South Carolina Vocational Rehabilitation Evaluation Center
1400 Boston Avenue | West Columbia, SC 29170
Tel: (803) 896-6047 | Fax: (803) 896-6148

Trident Senior Health Center
2070 Northbrook Blvd., Suite A-16 | Charleston, SC 29406
Tel: (843) 797-0416

William Jennings Bryan Dorn Veterans Affairs Medical Center
3602 Deerfield Drive | Columbia, SC 29204
Tel: (803) 776-4000 x6216 | Fax: (803) 695-7932

South Carolina Driving Regulations

Driver Licensing Agency
South Carolina Department of Public Safety | Department of Motor Vehicles
P.O. Box 1993 | Blythewood, SC 29016 | Tel: (803) 737-4000
Web site: www.scdps.org

Standard Length of license validation—10 years. Renewal options and conditions are done in person. Renewal by mail is permitted if there have been no violations in the past 2 years, and no suspensions, revocations, or cancellations. A vision test is required at time of renewal, and a written test is required only if the client has 5+ points on his/her record or if there appears to be a need. A road test is required only if there appears to be a need.

Age-based renewal procedures—5 years for drivers 65 and older. A vision test is required.

Reporting Procedures
  Physician/medical reporting   Permitted but not required
  Immunity   No

Legal protection	N/A
DMV *follow-up*	License is suspended upon referral and further examination is conducted.
*Other reporting	Will accept information from courts, other DMVs, and police.
Anonymity	N/A

Role of the Medical Advisory Board—The MAB determines the mental or physical fitness of license applicants through a medical evaluation process, and makes recommendations to the department's director or designee on the handling of impaired drivers.

South Carolina Driver Improvement Office | P.O. Box 1498 | Columbia, SC 29216

SOUTH DAKOTA

State Office on Aging

South Dakota Office of Adult Services & Aging—Department of Social Services
700 Governors Drive | Pierre, SD 57501
Tel: (605) 773-3656 | Fax: (605) 773-6834

Driver Rehabilitation and Assessment Programs

Avera Rehabilitation Associates
Avera Doctors Plaza 2 | 1100 East 21st Street, Suite 401
Sioux Falls, SD 57105 | Tel: (605) 322-7300 | Fax: (605) 322-7301

Aberdeen Rehabilitation Medicine
Physicians Plaza, Suite E201B | 201 South Lloyd Street
Aberdeen, SD 57401 | Tel: (605) 622-2898 | Fax: (605) 622-2896

Black Hills Rehab Hospital
120 Ponderosa, Box 306 | Hill City, SD 57745
Tel: (605) 574-3345 | Fax: (605) 539-9111

Valley Outpatient Rehabilitation and Sports Medicine
1210 West 18th Street | Sioux Falls, SD 57117 | Tel: (605) 333-4569

Yankton Regional Physical Medicine and Rehabilitation Center
1000 W 4th St., 5th Floor | Yankton, SD 57078 | Tel: (605) 668-8661

South Dakota Driving Regulations

Driver Licensing Agency
South Dakota Department of Public Safety | Office of Driver Licensing
118 West Capitol Avenue | Pierre, SD 57501
Tel: (800) 952-3696 or (605) 773-6883
Web site: www.state.sd.us/dcr/dl/sddriver.htm

Standard Length of license validation—5 years. Renewal options and conditions are done in person; renewal by mail for military and military dependents only. A vision test is required at time of renewal, however, a written and road test are not required at time of renewal.

Age-based renewal procedures—None

Reporting Procedures
　Physician/medical reporting　Physicians may report unsafe drivers if they so choose by submitting a "Request Re-Evaluation" form. The form can be found on the Office of Driver Licensing Web site
　Immunity　No
　DMV follow-up　An appointment is scheduled and the driver is notified to appear for an interview. A written test and road test may be required.

　Other reporting　Will accept information from courts, other DMVs, police, family members, and other sources.

　Anonymity　Not available

Role of the Medical Advisory Board—South Dakota does not have a medical advisory board. Medical information is reviewed by Department of Commerce & Regulation personnel. If the Department has good cause to believe that a licensed operator is not qualified to be licensed, it may upon written notice of at least 5 days require him or her to submit to an examination or interview. The Department shall take appropriate action, which may include suspending or revoking the license, permitting the individual to retain his/her license, or issuing a license subject to restrictions.

TENNESSEE

State Office on Aging

Tennessee Commission on Aging and Disability
Andrew Jackson Building | 500 Deaderick Street, No. 825
Nashville, TN 37243-0860 | Tel: (615) 741-2056 | Fax: (615) 741-3309

Driver Rehabilitation and Assessment Programs

AAA Driving Evaluation and Training
102 Timber Trail Drive | Lebanon, TN 37090
Tel: (615) 449-8998 | Fax: (615) 449-2520

Access Industries, Inc.
2509 Summer Avenue | Memphis, TN 38112-2627 | Tel: (901) 323-5438

Centennial Physical Rehabilitation Center
2300 Patterson Street | Nashville, TN 37203
Tel: (615) 342-1919 | Toll Free: (800) 242-5662

Fort Loudoun Therapy Center
Lenoir City, TN 37772 | Tel: (865) 271-6080 | Fax: (865) 271-6081

HEALTHSOUTH Cane Creek Rehabilitation Hospital
180 Mount Pelia Road | Martin, TN 38237 | Tel: (731) 587-4231

HEALTHSOUTH Chattanooga Rehabilitation Hospital
2412 McCallie Ave. | Chattanooga, TN 37404 | Tel: (423) 698-0221

Methodist Physical Therapy
991 Oak Ridge Turnpike | Oak Ridge, TN 37830
Tel: (865) 481-1198 | Fax: (865) 481-1049

511 West Central Avenue | LaFollette, TN 37766
Tel: (423) 562-1330 | Fax: (423) 562-7397

Mountain States Health Alliance, RehabPlus Center for Outpatient
Rehabilitation
RehabPlus—West Market | 1725 West Market Street
Tel: (423) 431-2840 | Fax: (423) 431-5548
Rehab Plus - James H, & Cecile C. Quillen Rehabilitation Hospital
2511 Wesley Street | Tel: (423) 952-1765 | Fax: (423) 283-9371
RehabPlus - Indian Path Medical Center | 2205 Pavilion Drive
Tel: (423) 857-7660 | Fax: (423) 857-7001
RehabPlus - Johnson County Health Center | 1901 South Shady Street
Tel: (423) 727- 1161 | Fax: (423) 727-1129

Nashville Rehabilitation Hospital
610 Gallatin Avenue | Nashville, TN 37206
Tel: (615) 226-4330 | Fax: (615) 650-0793

Occupational Rehabilitation Center of West Tennessee
67 American Drive | Jackson, TN 38301
Toll Free: (800) 235-9498 | Fax: (731) 427-8464

On The Road Evaluations & Training
180 Bradford Circle | Hendersonville, TN 37075
Tel: (615) 294-3825 | Fax: (615) 507-2059

Patricia Neal Rehabilitation Center
1901 Clinch Avenue | Knoxville, TN 37916
Tel: (865) 541-2493

Parkwest Therapy Center
9111 Executive Park Drive | Knoxville, TN 37923
Tel: (865) 694-3099 | Fax: (865) 539-6419
200 Fort Sanders West Blvd. | MOB-1, Suite 201 | Knoxville, TN 37922
Tel: (865) 531-5710 | Fax (865) 531-5704

Siskin Rehabilitation for Physical Rehabilitation
1 Siskin Plaza | Chattanooga, TN 37403
Tel: (423) 634-1646 | Fax: (423) 634-4578

The Driving Challenge
5830 Mt. Moriaha Extended, Suite 14
Memphis, TN 38115 | Tel: (901) 794-3631

Vanderbilt Bill Wilkerson Center
1114 19th Ave. South | Nashville, TN 37212
Tel: (615) 936-5045 | Fax: (615) 936-5063

World of Independence, Inc.
8742 Asheville Highway | Knoxville, TN 37924-4559
Tel: (865) 932-2880

Tennessee Driving Regulations

Driver Licensing Agency
Tennessee Department of Safety | Motor Vehicle Services
1150 Foster Avenue | Nashville, TN 37249 | Tel: (615) 741-3954
Web site: www.state.tn.us/safety

Standard Length of license validation—5 years. Renewal options and
conditions are done in person; mail and Internet renewal are permitted every
other cycle. There are no vision, written, or road tests at time of renewal.

Age-based renewal procedures—None

Reporting Procedures

Physician/medical reporting	Permitted but not required
Immunity	Yes
Legal protection	No
DMV follow-up	Driver is notified of referral in writing.
*Other reporting	Will accept information from courts, other DMVs, police, family members, and other sources.
Anonymity	Not available

Role of the Medical Advisory Board—The MAB is composed of volunteer
physicians, who review medical reports and make recommendations.

Actions are based upon the recommendation of the majority. Tel: (615) 251-5193

TEXAS

State Office on Aging

Texas Department of Aging & Disability Services
P.O. Box 149030 (W-619) | Austin, TX 78714-9030
Tel: (512) 438-3030 | Fax: (512) 438-4220

Driver Rehabilitation and Assessment Programs

Adaptive Driving Access, Inc.
3402 Lilac | Pasadena, TX 77505 | Tel: (281) 487-1969

Advanced Mobility Systems of Texas
2110 North Beach Street | Fort Worth, TX 76111 | Tel: (817) 429-1273

Baylor Institute for Rehabilitation
3505 Gaston Avenue | Dallas, TX 75246
Tel: (214) 820-9340 | Fax: (214) 820-9369

Chevron Texaco - Medical Services
1111 Bagby Street, Room 4298 | Houston, TX 77002
Tel: (713) 752-6137 | Fax: (713) 752-4652

Christus Santa Rosa Hospital - Outpatient Rehabilitation Services
2701 Babcock Road | San Antonio, TX 78229
Tel: (210) 705-6560 | Fax: (210) 705-6567

East Texas Medical Center - Rehabilitation Center
701 Olympic Plaza Circle | Tyler, TX 75701
Tel: (903) 596-3000 | Toll Free: (800) 338-7293

HEALTHSouth Medical Center
2124 Research Row | Dallas, TX 75235 | Tel: (214) 904-6575

Highlands Regional Rehabilitation Hospital
1395 George Dieter Drive | El Paso, TX 79936 | Tel: (915) 298-7222

Hillcrest Outpatient Rehabilitation
3320 Hillcrest Drive | Tel: (254) 202-2000

Houston Veteran Affairs Medical Center
24410 Norchester Way | Spring, TX 77389-3757 | Tel: (713) 794-7243

Mabee Rehabilitation Center
Richardson Tower - Harris Methodist Fort Worth Hospital
1301 Pennsylvania Avenue | Fort Worth, TX 76104
Tel: (817) 882-2760 | Toll Free: (866) 847-7342

Saint David's Rehabilitation
1005 E 32nd St. | Austin, TX 78705 | Tel: (512) 476-7111
Web site: http://www.stdavidsrehab.com

Senior Care Services | Presbyterian Hospital of Dallas
8200 Walnut Hill Lane | Dallas, TX 75231-4402 | Tel: (214) 345-6789

Strowmatt Rehabilitation Services, Inc.
11020 Old Katy Road, Suite 217 | Houston, TX 77043
Tel: (713) 722-0667 | Fax: (713) 722-0669

The Institute for Rehabilitation and Research (TIRR)
10907 I-10 East Freeway | Houston, Texas 77029-1911
Tel: (713) 674-2611 | Fax: (713) 674-3081
3440 Richmond Avenue | Houston, Texas 77046-3405
Tel: (713) 850-8472 | Fax (713) 850-8490
700 Town & Country Boulevard, Suite 2490
Houston, Texas 77024-4810 | Tel: (713) 722-0156 | Fax: (713) 722-7051
720 Ave. F North (Hwy. 60) | Bay City, TX 77414-3544
Tel: (979) 244-5562 | Fax (979) 244-5890
3512 Hwy. 365 | Nederland, TX 77627-7834
Tel: (409) 722-7246 | Fax: (409) 722-7450
3122 E Spencer Hwy. | Pasadena, TX 77504-1162
Tel: (713) 944-4144 | Fax: (713) 944-8302

University of Texas Health Center at Tyler—Rehabilitation Services
Department
11937 US Highway 271 | Tyler, TX 75708-3154.
Tel: (903) 877-7293 | Fax: (903) 877-5615

Wichita Valley Rehabilitation Hospital
302 Loop 11 | Wichita Falls, TX 76306 | Tel: (940) 397-8200

Wright Way Inc.
P.O. Box 460907 | Garland, TX 75046 | Tel: (972) 240-8839

Texas Driving Regulations

Driver Licensing Agency
Texas Department of Public Safety | Driver license Division
P.O. Box 4087 | Austin, TX 78773-0001
Tel: (512) 424-2967 or (512) 424-2602
Web site: www.txdps.state.tx.us

Standard Length of license validation—6 years. Renewal options and
conditions are done in person; if the client is eligible, renewal by Internet,
telephone, or mail is also available. A vision test is required at time of
renewal, however, there are no written or road test requirements.

Age-based renewal procedures—None

Reporting Procedures

Physician/medical reporting	Any physician licensed to practice medicine in the state of Texas may inform the Department of Public Safety with a signed letter. This release of information is an exception to the patient-physician privilege.
Immunity	Yes
Legal protection	Yes
DMV follow-up	The driver is notified in writing of the referral and required to provide medical information from his/her personal physician.
*Other reporting	Will accept information from courts, other DMVs, police, family members, and other sources
Anonymity	Not anonymous or confidential.

> However, an attempt is made to protect
> the identity of the reporter. If the client
> requests an administrative hearing, the
> identity of the reporter may be revealed
> at that time.

Role of the Medical Advisory Board—To advise the Department of Public
Safety on medical issues regarding individual drivers. The Department bases
its actions on the recommendation of the physician who reviews the case.
Texas Department of Public Safety | Medical Advisory Board
P.O. Box 4087 | Austin, TX 78773 | Tel: (512) 424-2344

UTAH

State Office on Aging

Utah Division of Aging & Adult Services - Department of Human
Services
120 North 200 West, Room 325 | Salt Lake City, UT 84103
Tel: (801) 538-3910 | Fax: (801) 538-4395

Driver Rehabilitation and Assessment Programs

American Fork Hospital - Physical Therapy and Outpatient Rehabilitation
Center
Tel: (801) 855-3438

Mountain West Physical Therapy - Cache Valley Specialty Hospital
2380 North 400 East | North Logan, UT 84341 | Tel: (435) 713-9700
451 West 600 North | Tremonton, UT 84337 | Tel: (435) 257-3809
1950 South Highway 89 | Perry, UT 84302 | Tel: (435) 723-1902
169 North Spring Creek Parkway Ste. 140
Providence, UT 84332 | Tel: (435) 755-8500

Salt Lake Regional Medical Center - The Quinney Rehabilitation
Institute
Tel: (801) 350-4111

University of Utah Health Science Center - Neuropsychiatric Institute
Clinical Assessment Center | 501 Chipeta Way | Salt Lake City, UT 84108
Tel: (801) 583-2500

Veteran Affairs Salt Lake City Health Care System
500 Foothill Drive | Salt Lake City, UT 84148
Tel: (801) 582-1565 | Toll Free: (800) 613-4012 | Fax: (801) 584-1289

Wasatch Peak Physical Therapy - Davis Hospital and Medical Center
1492 W Antelope Drive, Suite 100 | Layton, Utah 84041
Tel: (801) 825-8091

Utah Driving Regulations

Driver Licensing Agency
Utah Department of Public Safety | Driver License Division
P.O. Box 30560 | Salt Lake City, UT 84130-0560
Tel: (801) 965-4437 or (801) 965-3819
Web site: www.driverlicense.utah.gov

Standard Length of license validation—5 years. Renewal options and conditions are done in person; mail-in every other cycle if no suspensions, revocations, convictions, and not more than 4 violations. A vision test is required at time of renewal only for clients aged 65 and older. There is no written test for renewals and a road test is only required if the examiner feels the applicant's ability to drive is in question.

Age-based renewal procedures—Vision testing required at license renewal for clients aged 65 and older.

Reporting Procedures

Physician/medical reporting	Permitted but not required
Immunity	Any physician or person who becomes aware of a physical, mental or emotional impairment which appears to present an imminent threat to driving safety and reports this information to the Department of Public Safety in good faith shall have immunity from any damages claimed as a result of so doing.
Legal protection	No
DMV follow-up	Driver is notified in writing of referral. License is suspended upon referral.

*Other reporting	Will accept information from courts, other DMVs, police, family members, and other sources.
Anonymity	Not anonymous or confidential.

Role of the Medical Advisory Board—The MAB advises the Director of the Driver License Division and recommends written guidelines and standards for determining the physical, mental, and emotional capabilities appropriate to various types of driving in an effort to minimize the conflict between the individual's desire to drive and the community's desire for safety.

Utah Medical Advisory Board | University of Utah Hospital
Research Park | 615 Arapeen Drive, # 100 | Salt Lake City, UT 84108

VERMONT

State Office on Aging

Vermont Department of Aging and Disabilities
103 South Main Street, Osgood #1 | Waterbury, VT 05671-2301
Tel: (802) 241-2400 | Fax: (802) 241-2325

Driver Rehabilitation and Assessment Programs

Adaptive Driving Associates
226 Holiday Drive, Suite 31 | White River Junction, VT 50001
Tel: (802) 296-2004

Centers for Living and Rehabilitation
160 Hospital Drive | Bennington, VT 05201 | Tel: (802) 447-5466

Central Vermont Medical Center Geriatric Rehabilitation Program
Medical Office Building A, 2nd Floor | 130 Fisher Road,
Berlin, VT 05642 | Tel: (802) 371-4242 | Fax: (802) 371-5350

Driver Rehabilitation Institute
5A David Drive | Essex Jct., VT 05452
Fax: (802) 879-5334 | Web site: www.DRIVermont.com

32 Grant Street | Burlington, VT 05401
Tel: (802) 876-1800 x25 | Fax: (802) 879-5334

Porter Rehabilitation and Orthopedic Services (PROS)
115 Porter Drive | Middlebury, VT 05753 | Tel: (802) 388-4777

Rutland Regional Medical Center - Rehabilitation Services
160 Allen Street | Rutland, VT 05701
Tel: (802) 5-7111 | Fax: (802) 747-1620

Southwestern Vermont Medical Center - Outpatient Rehabilitation
Department
Toolan Building | 120 Hospital Drive | Bennington, VT 05201
Tel: (802) 447-5140

Springfield Hospital - Rehabilitation Services
441 River Street | North Springfield, VT 05150 | Tel: (802) 886-2172

Vermont Driving Regulations

Driver Licensing Agency
Vermont Agency of Transportation | Department of Motor Vehicles
120 State Street | Montpelier, VT 05603-0001 | Tel: (802) 828-2000
Web site: www.aot.state.vt.us

Standard Length of license validation—4 years. Renewal options and
conditions are done by mail or in person. There are no vision, written, or
road tests required at time of renewal.

Age-based renewal procedures—None

Reporting Procedures

Physician/medical reporting	Physicians may provide information to the DMV only with the permission of the patient.
Immunity	No
Legal protection	No
DMV follow-up	Driver is notified of the referral by mail.

| *Other reporting | Will accept information from courts, other DMVs, police, concerned citizens, or family members. The letter must be signed. |

| Anonymity | Not anonymous or confidential. However, the reporter's identity is held confidential until a hearing is requested by the client. |

Role of the Medical Advisory Board—Vermont no longer retains a medical advisory board.

VIRGINIA

State Office on Aging

Virginia Department for the Aging
1610 Forest Avenue, Suite 100 | Richmond, VA 23229
Tel: (804) 662-9333 | Fax: (804) 662-9354

Driver Rehabilitation and Assessment Programs

Alert Driver Training of Vinton
P.O. Box 1176 | Vinton, VA 24179 | Tel: (540) 890-0347

Bedford Memorial Hospital - Rehabilitation Services and Geriatric Services
1613 Oakwood St. | P.O. Box 688 | Bedford, VA 24523
Tel: (540) 586-2441

Bon Secours Hampton Roads Health System - Senior Health Services
On-Road Certified Driving Clinic
DePaul Medical Center: (757) 889-5976
Mary Immaculate Hospital: (757) 886-6700
Maryview Medical Center: (757) 398-2273

Boundless Mobility
73 Pheasant Run | Waynesboro, VA 22980 | Tel: (540) 943-3898

Centra Health Rehabilitation Services
Virginia Baptist Hospital: (434) 947-4668
Lynchburg General Hospital: (434) 947-3037
Guggenheimer Nursing Home: (434) 947-7425
Centra Health Medical Center-Gretna: (434) 947-5439

Johnston-Willis Hospital Driver Education and Training Program
1401 Johnston Willis Drive | Occupational Therapy First Floor
Richmond, VA 23235 | Tel: (804) 330-2068 | Fax: (804) 330-2144

Lewis-Gale Outpatient Rehabilitation Services
1902 Braeburn Drive | Salem, VA 24153 | Tel: (540) 772-2816
6701 Peters Creek Road, Suite 105 | Roanoke, VA 24019
Tel: (540) 563-8462

Mobility Center of Virginia
249-255 E German School Road | Richmond, VA 23224
Tel: (804) 231-7774

Riverside Rehabilitation Institute
245 Chesapeake Avenue | Newport News, VA 23607
Tel: (757) 928-8363 | Fax: (757) 928-8108

Roanoke Memorial Hospital, Carilion Center for Healthy Aging
Geriatric Assessment | 1906 Belleview Avenue | P.O. Box 13367
Roanoke, VA 24033 | Tel: (540) 981-7000

Sheltering Arms Physical Rehabilitation Hospital
8254 Atlee Road | Mechanicsville, VA 23116 | Tel: (804) 342-4100

Veteran Affairs Medical Center Hampton Virginia
63 Brogden Lane | Hampton, VA 23666
Tel: (757) 722-9961 x2202 | Fax: (757) 728-3455

University of Virginia Disability Evaluation Services
545 Ray C. Hunt Drive, Suite 310 | Charlottesville, VA 22908-1007
Tel: (434) 243-5622 or (434) 243-5639

University of Virginia Physical Medicine & Rehabilitation
Neurocognitive Assessment | 545 Ray C. Hunt Drive, Suite 240
Box 801004 | Charlottesville, VA 22908-1004
Tel: (434) 924-2718 | Fax: (434) 243-6546

University of Virginia HEALTHSOUTH Rehabilitation Hospital
515 Ray C. Hunt Drive | Charlottesville, VA 22903 | Tel: (434) 244-2000

Woodrow Wilson Rehabilitation Center | Box W476 | P.O. Box 1500
Fishersville, VA 22939 | Tel: (540) 332-7117 | Fax: (540) 332-7194

Winchester Rehabilitation Center
333 W Cork Street | Winchester, VA 22601
Tel: (540) 536-5113 | Fax: (540) 665-5139

Virginia Driving Regulations

Driver Licensing Agency
Virginia Department of Motor Vehicles | P.O. Box 27212
Richmond, VA 23269 | Tel: (866) 368-5463 | Web site: www.dmv.state.va.us

Standard Length of license validation—5 years. For renewal options and
conditions customers may use an alternative method of renewing their
driver's license every other cycle unless their license has been suspended or
revoked, they have 2 or more violations, there is a DMV medical review
indicator on the license, or they fail the vision test. Alternative methods
include mail-in, Internet, touch-tone telephone, fax, and ExtraTeller. There
is a vision test at time of renewal and a written test is required if the customer
has had 2 or more violations in the past 5 years. A road test is not required.

Age-based renewal procedures—None

Reporting Procedures
  Physician/medical reporting   Physicians are not required to report
                                         unsafe drivers. However, for physicians
                                         who do report unsafe drivers, laws have
                                         been enacted to prohibit release of the
                                         physician's name as the source of the
                                         report.

Immunity	No
Legal protection	Va Code ß 54 1-2966 1 states that if a physician reports a patient to the DMV, it shall not constitute a violation of the doctor-patient relationship unless the physician has acted with malice.
DMV follow-up	Drivers are notified in writing that the DMV has initiated a medical review and advised of the medical review requirements. Drivers are also advised of any restrictions or suspension imposed as a result of the review.
*Other reporting	The DMV relies upon information from courts, other DMVs, law enforcement officers, physicians, and other medical professionals, relatives, and concerned citizens to help identify drivers who may be impaired.
Anonymity	Not anonymous. Virginia law provides confidentiality, but only for relatives and physicians.

Role of the Medical Advisory Board—The MAB enables the DMV to monitor drivers throughout the state who may have physical or mental problems. The MAB assists the Commissioner with the development of medical and health standards for use in the issuance of driver's licenses. The MAB helps the DMV avoid the issuance of licenses to persons suffering from any physical or mental disability or disease that will prevent their exercising reasonable and ordinary control over a motor vehicle while driving it on highways. The MAB reviews the more complex cases, including those referred for administrative hearings, and provides recommendations for medical review action.

Virginia Department of Motor Vehicles | Medical Review Services
P.O. Box 27412 | Richmond, VA 23269
Tel: (804) 367-0531 | Fax: (804) 367-1604

WASHINGTON

State Office on Aging

Washington Aging and Disability Services
Department of Social & Health Services | Mail Stop 45050
14th and Jefferson, Office Bldg. 2 | Olympia, WA 98504-5010
Tel: (360) 902-7797 | Fax: (360) 902-7848

Driver Rehabilitation and Assessment Programs

Auburn Regional Medical Center, Rehabilitation Center–Outpatient Clinic
202 North Division St. | Auburn, WA 98001
Tel: (253) 804-2823 | Fax: (253) 804-2831

Kirshner Driving School
6800 48th Avenue NE | Seattle, WA 98115
Tel: (206) 524-4823 | Fax: (206) 526-7368

Good Samaritan Older Adult Services
407 14th Ave. SE | Puyallup, WA 98372 | Tel: (253) 435-7253

Harborview Medical Center SeniorCare Clinic
Tel: (206) 731-4191 | Fax: (206) 531-8527

Holy Family Hospital - Rehabilitation Services
5633 N Lidgerwood | Spokane, WA 99208 | Tel: (509) 482-0111

Northwoods Ledge
2321 Schold Place | Silverdale, WA 98346 | Tel: (360) 337-7422

PROVAIL
3670 Stone Way N | Seattle, WA 98103-8004
Tel: (206) 826-1045 | Fax: (206) 826-1145

Providence Everett Medical Center
916 Pacific Avenue | Everett, WA 98206-1067
Tel: (425) 258-7847 | Fax: (425) 258-7136

St. Lukes Rehabilitation Institute
17514 E Bill Gulch Road | Mead, WA 99021
Tel: (509) 238-2580 or (509) 838-4771

Swedish Medical Center - Outpatient Rehabilitation Center
Ballard campus: (206) 781-6346
First Hill campus: (206) 386-2035
Providence campus: (206) 320-2404
West Seattle Clinic: (206) 320-5510

University. of Washington Medical Center
11521 Fremont Avenue N | Seattle, WA 98133
Tel: (206) 598-4833 or (206) 598-5857 | Fax: (206) 598-4897

Washington Driving Regulations

Driver Licensing Agency
Washington Department of Licensing | Driver Services
1125 Washington Street SE | P.O. Box 9020 | Olympia, WA 98507-9020
Tel: (360) 902-3600 | Web site: www.dol.wa.gov

Standard Length of license validation—5 years. For renewal options and
conditions: in-state renewals are in person only. If out of state, the
applicant can renew by mail once. A vision test is required at time of
renewal, and a written and road test are required only if warranted by
results of vision, health, or medical screening.

Age-based renewal procedures—None

Reporting Procedures
Physician/medical reporting	Permitted but not required
Immunity	No
Legal protection	No
DMV follow-up	The DMV sends a letter to the driver with information detailing due process and action following any failure to respond.
*Other reporting	Will accept information from courts, other DMVs, police, family members, and other competent sources. If in doubt, the reporting party may be required to establish his/her firsthand knowledge and standing for making a report.

Anonymity   Not anonymous or confidential.

Role of the Medical Advisory Board—Washington does not retain a medical advisory board.

WEST VIRGINIA

State Office on Aging

West Virginia Bureau of Senior Services
1900 Kanawha Boulevard East | 3003 Town Center Mall
Charleston, WV 25305-0160 | Tel: (304) 558-3317 | Fax: (304) 558-5609

Driver Rehabilitation and Assessment Programs

Broaddus Hospital - Physical Therapy and Rehabilitation
Mansfield Hill 119 South | Philippi, WV 26416
Tel: (304) 457-1760

Hanshaw Geriatric Center
1600 Medical Center Drive | Huntington, WV 25701
Tel: (304) 526-2078 | Fax: (304) 733-4208

HEALTHSOUTH Rehabilitation Hospital Huntington
6900 W Country Club Drive | Huntington, WV 25705
Tel: (304) 733-1060 | Fax: (304) 733-4208

St. Mary's Medical Center
2900 1st Ave. | Huntington, WV 25702
Tel: (304) 526-1334 | Fax: (304) 526-1335

Thomas Memorial Hospital - Physical Therapy Center
4605 MacCorkle Avenue SW | South Charleston, WV 25309
Tel: (304) 766-3589

United Rehabilitation
600 Davisson Run Road, Suite 101 | Tel: (304) 623-2330
1221 Johnson Avenue, Suite 1000 | Bridgeport, WV 26330
Tel: (304) 842-3898

West Virginia Rehabilitation Center - Driver Education Department
P.O. Box 1004 | Institute, WV 25112-1004
Tel: (304) 766-4745 | Fax: (304) 766-4923

West Virginia School of Medicine - The Bradford B. Laidley 65Plus Clinic
P.O. Box 9897 | Stadium Drive | Morgantown, WV 26507
Tel: (304) 598-4850 | Fax: (304) 598-4871

West Virginia Driving Regulations

Driver Licensing Agency
West Virginia Department of Transportation | Division of Motor
Vehicles
Building 3, Room 113 | 1800 Kanawha Boulevard East
Charleston WV 25317
Tel: (800) 642-9066 or (304) 558-3900 | Web site: www.wvdot.com

Standard Length of license validation—5 years. Under the "Drive for Five"
program, all driver's licenses expire in the client's birth month at an age
divisible by five (e.g., 25, 30, 35, etc). Renewal options and conditions: In
person. There is no vision, written or road testing required at time of
renewal.

Age-based renewal procedures—None

Reporting Procedures

Physician/medical reporting	Physicians are permitted and encouraged to report.
Immunity	No
Legal protection	No
DMV *follow-up*	A medical report is sent to the driver, to be completed by his/her physician. If the driver fails to comply, then the driver's license is immediately revoked.
*Other reporting	Will accept information from law enforcement officers and family members.
Anonymity	Not anonymous or confidential.

Role of the Medical Advisory Board—If the MAB concludes that the driver is unsafe, it may recommend to the Commissioner of Motor Vehicles that the license be revoked. The Commissioner then makes the final licensing decision.
Tel: (304) 558-0238

WISCONSIN

State Office on Aging

Wisconsin Bureau of Aging and LTC Resources
Department of Health and Family Services
One West Wilson Street, Room 450 | P.O. Box 7851
Madison, WI 53707-7851
Tel: (608) 266-2536 | Fax: (608) 267-3203

Driver Rehabilitation and Assessment Programs

Drive Safe Midwest
4737 N Elkhart Avenue | Milwaukee, WI 53211 | Tel: (414) 688-1081

Elmbrook Memorial Hospital
19333 W North Avenue | Brookfield, WI 53045 | Tel: (262) 785-2187

Gundersen Lutheran
1910 South Avenue | LaCrosse, WI 54601 | Tel: (608) 782-7300 x40

Meriter Hospital
202 S Park Street | Madison, WI 53715 | Tel: (608) 267-6173

North Chicago Veteran Affairs Hospital
980 Rhyners Lane | Twin Lakes, WI 53181 | Tel: (847) 688-1900

Rehab Plus
P.O. Box 1450 | Manitowoc, WI 54221-9950 | Tel: (920) 686-3100

Sacred Heart Rehabilitation
2350 N Lake Drive | Milwaukee, WI 53211 | Tel: (414) 298-6798

Southwest Health Center
Mood and Memory Screening | 1400 East Side Road
Platteville, WI 53818 | Tel: (608) 744-3156

St. Mary's Hospital
13111 N Port Washington Road | Mequon, WI 53097 | Tel: (262) 243-7444

St. Mary's Ozaukee
13111 N Port Washington Road | Mequon, WI 53092 | Tel: (414) 351-8850

St. Michael's Hospital - Physical Therapy Department
2400 W Villard | Milwaukee, WI 53209 | Tel: (414) 527-8000

St. Vincent Hospital - Occupational Therapy Department
835 S Van Buren | Green Bay, WI 54301 | Tel: (920) 433-8693

Theda Clark Medical Center - Occupational Therapy Department
130 Second Street | Neenah, WI 54956 | Tel: (920) 729-3100

University of Wisconsin Hospital and Clinics - Memory Assessment
Clinic
600 Highland Ave. | Madison, WI 53792 | Tel: (608) 263-7740

University of Wisconsin Hospital and Clinics - Geriatrics Clinics
5249 E Terrace Dr. | Madison, WI 53718 | Tel: (608) 265-1210
451 Junction Rd. | Madison, WI 53717 | Tel: (608) 263-5010
6209 Mineral Point Road | Madison, WI 53705 | Tel: (608) 231-0757

University Station Clinic - Mobility and Falls Clinic
2880 University Ave. | Madison, WI 53705 | Tel: (608) 263-7740

Wisconsin Driving Regulations

Driver Licensing Agency
Wisconsin Department of Transportation | Bureau of Driver Services
Hill Farm State Transportation Building | 4802 Sheboygan Avenue
P.O. Box 7910 | Madison, WI 53707-7910 | Tel: (608) 266-2353
Web site: www.dot.wisconsin.gov

Standard Length of license validation—8 years. Renewal options and conditions are done in person; by mail if client is out of state. There is a vision test at time of renewal. A written and road test is determined by DOT, vision specialist, or physician.

Age-based renewal procedures—None

Reporting Procedures

Physician/medical reporting	Physicians are encouraged though not required to report. They can report by submitting form MV3141 ("Driver Condition or Behavior Report") or a letter on letterhead stationery. Form MV3141 is available on the DOT Web site.
Immunity	Yes
Legal protection	Yes
DMV follow-up	Driver is notified in writing of requirement(s). Depending on requirement(s), he/she is given 15, 30, or 60 days to comply. If driver does not comply within the time period given, the driver's license is cancelled. Driver is notified in writing of cancellation.
*Other reporting	Will accept information from courts, other DMVs, police, family members, and other sources.
Anonymity	Not anonymous or confidential (Wisconsin has an Open Records Law). However, individuals can submit "Pledge of Confidentiality" form MV3454 with form MV3141 Form MV3454 is available on the DOT Web site.

Role of the Medical Advisory Board—The MAB advises the Bureau of Driver Services on medical issues regarding individual drivers. Wisconsin has 2 types of MAB:

1. By-Mail-Board: paper file is mailed to 3 physicians specialists (i.e., neurologist, endocrinologist, ophthalmologist) for recommendations based on the client's medical condition(s).

2. In-Person Board: the client has an interview with 3 physicians (psychiatrist, neurologist, and internist). Actions are based on the recommendation of the majority, the client's driving record, medical information provided by the client's physician and, if appropriate, driving examination results.

WYOMING

State Office on Aging

Wyoming Aging Division - Department of Health
6101 Yellow Stone Road | Room 259B | Cheyenne, WY 82002
Tel: (307) 777-7986 or (800) 442-2766 | Fax: (307) 777-5340

Driver Rehabilitation and Assessment Programs

Castle Rock Hospital District - Occupational Therapy
1400 Uinta Drive | Green River, WY 82935
Tel: (307) 872-4526 | Fax: (307) 872-4595

Evanston Regional Hospital - Rehabilitation Services
190 Arrowhead Drive | Evanston, WY 82930
Physical Therapy: (307) 783-8220
Occupational Therapy: (307) 783-8220

Ivinson Memorial Hospital - Physical & Occupational Therapy
255 North 30th Street | Laramie, WY 82072 | Tel: (307) 742-2141 x2437

North Big Horn Hospital District - Occupational Therapy
1115 Lane 12 | Lovell, WY 82431 | Tel: (307) 548-5231

North Platte Physical Therapy
P.O. Box 1790 | Douglas, WY 82633 | Tel: (307) 358-9464

St. John's Medical Center - Rehabilitation
P.O. Box 428 | 625 E Broadway | Jackson, WY 83001 |Tel: (307) 739-7626

West Park Hospital - Rehabilitation Services
707 Sheridan Ave. | Cody, WY 82414 | Tel: (307) 578-2452

Wyoming Orthopedic and Rehabilitation Institute
Tel: (307) 688-8000

Wyoming Driving Regulations

Driver Licensing Agency
Wyoming Department of Transportation | Driver Services
5300 Bishop Boulevard | Cheyenne, WY 82009-3340
Tel: (307) 777-4800 or (307) 777-4810 | Web site: www.dot.state.wy.us

Standard Length of license validation—4 years. Renewal options and
conditions are done in person; mail-in every other cycle. A vision test is
required at time of renewal. A written test is not required at time of
renewal, but a road test is required only if warranted by a vision statement
from physician or examiner.

Age-based renewal procedures—None

Reporting Procedures

Physician/medical reporting	Physician reporting is encouraged, though not required.
Immunity	Physicians providing information concerning a patient's ability to drive safely are immune from liability for their opinions and recommendations.
Legal protection	N/A
DMV follow-up	If necessary, the DOT obtains additional information from the physician through completion of a Driver Medical Evaluation form.
Other reporting	Will accept information from courts, other DMVs, police, and family members.
Anonymity	N/A

Role of the Medical Advisory Board—Wyoming does not retain a medical
advisory board.

American Geriatrics Society, 136
American Heart Association (AHA),
 76
American Medical Association
 (AMA), 4, 16, 38, 70, 140
American Occupational Therapy,
 140–41
American Public Transportation
 Association, 140
American Society on Aging, 135
Americans with Disabilities Act, 90
anger, 86–87
angina, 31
antibiotics, 53–54
anticholinergics, 42–43
anticonvulsants, 43–44
antidepressants, 44–45
antiemetics, 45
antihistamines, 45–46
antihypertensives, 46–47
antipsychotics, 47
anxiety, 35–36, 43, 47, 86
Arizona, resources and driving
 regulations for, 149–51
Arkansas, resources and driving
 regulations for, 151–52
arthritis, 33–34, 49
articles, guides, booklets, and
 handbooks, 144–45
assessment of driving fitness, 1–19
 age and, 3–4
 cognitive, 13–14, 15–16, 17–18
 by driving rehabilitation specialist,
  18–19
 driving skill, 14
 forms, 123–27
 by healthcare provider, 16–18
 home, 14–16
 mobility, 14, 15–16, 18

planning to avoid dilemmas and,
 60–65
vision, 13, 15–16, 17
warning signs of driving risk,
 4–12
Assessment of Driving-Related Skills
 (ADReS), 17–18
assistive devices, 120–22
Association for Driver Rehabilitation
 Specialists, 134
Ativan, 47
attention, 13–14
 problems, 13, 28–29
attention deficit/hyperactivity
 disorder (ADHD), 50
attorney, 71–72
 power of, 72–74
automobile industry, xvi
 advertising, xvi

Benadryl, 46
benzodiazepines (sedatives), 47–48
Beverly Foundation, 141
bipolar disorder, 43
blindness, 26
brain disorders, xv–xvi, 28–29; *see
 also* dementia
brakes, pumping, 11
breast cancer, 21
Brown, Todd, 80, 81
Bureau of Transportation Statistics,
 138

California, resources and driving
 regulations for, 152–56
cancer, 3, 21
car, 2
 advertising, xvi
 crashes, xiii, xv, 5